HIPAA Compliance in Health Care

Security and Management of Health Information

Compiled by Christopher Miller DHSc

Keiser University

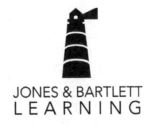

JONES & BARTLETT
L E A R N I N G

World Headquarters
Jones & Bartlett Learning
5 Wall Street
Burlington, MA 01803
978-443-5000
info@jblearning.com
www.jblearning.com

Jones & Bartlett Learning books and products are available through most bookstores and online booksellers. To contact Jones & Bartlett Learning directly, call 800-832-0034, fax 978-443-8000, or visit our website, www.jblearning.com.

This book is produced through PUBLISH – a custom publishing service offered by Jones & Bartlett Learning. For more information on PUBLISH, contact us at 800-832-0034 or visit our website at www.jblearning.com.

Disclaimer
This publication is sold with the understanding that the publisher is not engaged in rendering medical, legal, accounting, or other professional services. If medical, legal, accounting, or other professional service advice is required, the service of a competent professional should be sought. The authors, editor, and publisher have designed this publication to provide accurate information with regard to the subject matter covered. However, they are not responsible for errors, omissions, or for any outcomes related to the use of the contents of this publication and make no guarantee and assume no responsibility or liability for the use of the products and procedures described, or the correctness, sufficiency, or completeness of stated information, opinions, or recommendations. Treatments and side effects described in this publication are not applicable to all people; required dosages and experienced side effects will vary among individuals. Drugs and medical devices discussed herein are controlled by the Food and Drug Administration (FDA) and may have limited availability for use only in research studies or clinical trials. Research, clinical practice, and government regulations often change accepted standards. When consideration is being given to the use of any drug in the clinical setting, the health care provider or reader is responsible for determining FDA status of the drug, reading the package insert, and reviewing prescribing information for the most current recommendations on dose, precautions, and contraindications and for determining the appropriate usage for the product. This is especially important in the case of drugs that are new or seldom used. Any references in this publication to procedures to be employed when rendering emergency care to the sick and injured are provided solely as a general guide; other or additional safety measures might be required under particular circumstances. This publication is not intended as a statement of the standards of care required in any particular situation; circumstances and the physical conditions of patients can vary widely from one emergency to another. This publication is not intended in any way to advise emergency personnel concerning their legal authority to perform the activities or procedures discussed. Such local determination should be made only with the aid of legal counsel. Some images in this publication feature models; these models do not necessarily endorse, represent, or participate in the activities represented in the images.

Cover Image: © Photos.com

6048
Printed in the United States of America
24 23 22 21 20   36 35 34 33 32

Contents

Healthcare Information

Joan M. Lebow, JD, Joseph L. Ternullo, JD, MPH, Cavan K. Doyle, JD, LLM, Cheryl A. Miller, JD, and Kelly L. Gawne, JD

Key Learning Objectives

By the end of this chapter, the reader will be able to:

- Understand some of the legal issues related to the collection, use, and disclosure of healthcare information.

- Identify some of the underlying issues concerning healthcare information, ownership of the information, requirements about content, privacy requirements, and uses and disclosure of healthcare information.

- Appreciate a wide range of federal and state laws governing the use and disclosure of healthcare information and the security of such information.

- Understand some of the threats to the security of healthcare information in the context of digital media and the Internet.

Chapter Outline

1. What are the underlying issues addressed through the laws concerning healthcare information?

2. Who owns medical records?

3. What records must be created, and how must they be maintained?

4. What are the laws concerning privacy of healthcare information?

5. What are the laws concerning use of healthcare information?

6. What are the laws concerning disclosure of healthcare information?

7. What legal issues flow from the use of audio and video transmissions and recordings?

8. What legal issues flow from the use of computers and the Internet?

Introduction

The collection, use, and disclosure of healthcare information have become some of the most heavily regulated areas of health care. Healthcare providers must record, generate, and handle a large amount of information. This includes sensitive information about patients that is necessary to provide treatment. It also includes a wide range of information that is required for business and other internal operations, payment, and regulatory purposes.

Providers and others who obtain healthcare information need to be aware of the applicable requirements when collecting, using, and disclosing healthcare information. The details of these requirements are beyond the scope of this book.

This chapter addresses the following questions:

- 1. What are the underlying issues addressed through the laws concerning healthcare information?
- 2. Who owns medical records?
- 3. What records must be created, and how must they be maintained?
- 4. What are the laws concerning privacy of healthcare information?
- 5. What are the laws concerning use of healthcare information?
- 6. What are the laws concerning disclosure of healthcare information?
- 7. What legal issues flow from the use of audio and video transmissions and recordings?
- 8. What legal issues flow from the use of computers and the Internet?

1 What Are the Underlying Issues Addressed Through the Laws Concerning Healthcare Information?

Laws dealing with the use and disclosure of healthcare information seek to address a wide spectrum of troublesome issues. Such problems include: (1) balancing patient concerns for confidentiality with the need for access to healthcare information and the cost of implementing confidentiality protections; (2) balancing accountability for healthcare services with the cost to satisfy documentation requirements; (3) addressing government and business desires to access information for a wide variety of purposes ranging from law enforcement to budgeting to marketing; (4) managing the sharing of electronic health information across healthcare provider networks; (5) aggregating health information to facilitate research and improve health outcomes; and (6) implementing sanctions and penalties for unauthorized disclosure of health information.

PROVIDING HEALTHCARE SERVICES. Healthcare providers must access, collect, and use healthcare information to provide healthcare services. Specifically, providers use medical records and other types of health information as communication tools in caring for patients with healthcare problems. Patients are often treated by several different providers in multiple different treatment settings. As such, providers must exchange patient information to provide continuity of care. Electronic health records are becoming increasingly prevalent in response to the demand for instant access to information about patients' past and present health conditions and treatment and incentives provided under federal law—the American Relief and Recovery Act of 2009 (ARRA). It provides billions of dollars for health information technology investments. Most of the money is available to hospitals and physicians who adopt and meaningfully use qualified electronic health records. The vision and objective is that these qualifying electronic health records will enable providers to quickly and easily access patient information across diverse treatment settings, thus improving continuity in patient care.

CONFIDENTIALITY. A physician has a duty to protect the confidential health information of his or her patient. The purpose of the duty of confidentiality is to encourage patients to make a full and frank disclosure of information to the physician. Full disclosure enables the physician to diagnose conditions accurately and to provide appropriate treatment to further protect their privacy, patients may seek to limit who, outside of the doctor-patient relationship, has access to their confidential health information. However, the patient's interest in keeping his medical information private may conflict with other entities' interest in accessing the information. For example, an employer may seek information about a potential employee's tobacco use or other health habits, or an insurance company may require a medical exam and information about preexisting health conditions before issuing a health insurance policy. The conflict between the individual's desire to maintain the confidentiality of his or her health information and society's countervailing desire or ability to discover it is at the heart of many of the current debates in healthcare law.

ACCOUNTABILITY. Documentation of patient care and the medical services provided to patients is critical in maintaining provider accountability. Each step of a patient's encounter with a medical professional is documented, through, for example, notations in the patient's medical record, correspondence between the provider and the insurance company, and entries in a pharmacy's computer system. In the event of an adverse event in the patient's care, debate over payment of a provider's bill, or other problem, the collected documentation serves as the primary source of information in determining accountability. To this end, healthcare information and documentation may be used for internal quality review, medical negligence and malpractice liability lawsuits, and regulatory and accreditation requirements.

USES OF INFORMATION FOR OTHER PURPOSES. Individuals, healthcare providers, private businesses, government agencies, and other entities seek access to identifiable healthcare information for a wide range of purposes, including:

1. Performance improvement (finding ways to improve services);

2. Clinical research (advancing medical knowledge and practice);

3. Public health and safety (e.g., protecting from contagious diseases);

4. Billing and collections (justifying payment);

5. Planning and marketing by healthcare providers;

6. Documenting individuals' conditions (e.g., to be excused from specific duties[1] and to make benefits and other legal claims);

7. Law enforcement (e.g., to investigate and prove crimes);

8. Government planning;

9. Media reporting; and

10. Other business uses (e.g., building databases for marketing and planning).[2]

2 Who Owns Medical Records?

The hospital or other healthcare institution owns the medical record, which is its business record. Institutional ownership is explicitly stated in the statutes and regulations of some states, and courts have recognized this ownership.[3] If a physician has separate records, they are the physician's property, but the physician is still responsible for maintaining complete institutional records.

The medical record is an unusual type of property because, physically, it belongs to the institution and the institution must exercise considerable control over access, but the patient and others have an interest in the information in the record. The institution owns the paper or other material on which the information is recorded,[4] but it has responsibilities concerning access to and use and disclosure of the information. The patient and others have a right of access to the information in many circumstances, but they do not have a right to possession of original records.[5] Courts have ruled that patients do not have a right to pathology slides[6] or x-ray negatives.[7] The patient does not purchase a picture; the patient purchases the professional service of interpreting the x-ray. Thus, the patient could not use the physician's retention of the x-ray as a defense to a suit to collect professional fees.

The institutional medical record belongs to the institution. While associated with the institution, physicians and other individual providers have access to the records for patient care, administrative uses, and some legal purposes.[8] After physicians or other providers no longer have association with the institution, they have more limited access but generally can obtain access for legal purposes, for example, defending lawsuits and administrative proceedings or collecting bills. However, individual providers generally are not custodians of the records. Subpoenas and other efforts to discover institutional records should be directed to the institutional custodian, not the individual provider.

Ownership issues sometimes arise between providers, especially when physicians are terminated from employment. The outcomes vary depending on state law and what the employment agreement says.[9]

3 What Records Must Be Created, and How Must They Be Maintained?

Healthcare providers are required by both governmental and nongovernmental organizations (NGOs) to have accurate and complete medical records. The licensing laws and regulations of many states include specific requirements with which hospitals and other providers must comply. In addition, nongovernmental agencies, such as The Joint Commission (TJC), establish medical records standards.

The primary purpose of medical records is to facilitate diagnosis, treatment, and patient care. Records provide a communications link among the team members caring for the patient. Records also document what was found and what was done so that patient care can be evaluated, billing and collections can be performed, and other administrative and legal matters can be addressed. Medical records are also valuable in hospital educational and research programs.

This section addresses:

- 3.1. What elements must healthcare records contain?
- 3.2. Why must medical records be accurate, timely, and legible?
- 3.3. How should corrections and alterations in records be handled?
- 3.4. How long should records be retained, and how should they be destroyed?

3.1 What Elements Must Healthcare Records Contain?

Many statutes and regulations require healthcare providers to maintain medical records. Healthcare providers that participate in Medicare must comply with minimum content requirements.[10] Some local governments require additional information to be kept. Billing requirements of other payers also add requirements.

To be accredited, hospitals must meet the TJC's medical records standards, including a long list of items that must be in the medical record to assure identification of the patient, support for the diagnosis, justification for the treatment, and accurate documentation of results.[11] While some items apply only to inpatients, the general standards apply to all patients.

Individual healthcare providers can lose their licenses for failure to maintain required records.[12]

The medical record consists of three types of data: (1) personal, (2) financial, and (3) medical.

Personal information, usually obtained upon admission, includes name, date of birth, sex, marital status, occupation, other items of identification, and the next of kin or other contact person. The accuracy of this information often depends on the knowledge and honesty of the person providing the information. Providers can generally rely on the information provided unless there is significant reason to doubt it. In 1998, a New York court ruled that a hospital could rely on information provided on a patient's behalf, so it was proper to serve a collection action at the address given by an adult patient's father when she was admitted.[13]

Financial data usually include the patient's employer, health insurance identification, and other information to assist billing.

Medical data forms the clinical record, a continuously maintained history of patient condition and treatment, including physical examinations, medical history, treatment administered, progress reports, physician orders, clinical laboratory reports, radiology reports, consultation reports, anesthesia records, operation records, signed consent forms, nursing notes, and discharge summaries. The medical record should be a complete, current record of the history, condition, and treatment of the patient.

Incomplete hospital recordkeeping can sometimes be used to infer negligence in treatment.[14] One federal court found a hospital negligent for permitting its nurse to chart by exception in postoperative monitoring.[15] Minor variations from hospital standards concerning charting do not automatically prove that an examination or treatment did not meet legal standards. A federal court found that an emergency screening satisfied the law even though the full hospital screening procedure was not followed.[16]

Governmental and private third-party payers and managed care organizations are demanding that an increased amount of information be documented to justify treatment, referral, or payment.[17] This is changing the nature of medical practice and diverting clinical time and institutional resources to comply with these requirements.

CODING. Medicare and most managed care companies require providers to code their services, which means that a number must be assigned to each service from a complex coding system. Generally, provider records must include documentation of the diagnosis and treatment to support the coding.

Due to the complexity and changing nature of the coding systems and the liability for coding errors, most institutional providers have had to hire professional coders to assign the codes on each bill.

3.2 Why Must Medical Records Be Accurate, Timely, and Legible?

Accurate and timely completion of medical records is essential to maximizing availability of information for treatment, expediting payment, complying with governmental and accreditation requirements, and minimizing liability exposure.

State licensing statutes and regulations and TJC standards require accurate records.[18] An inaccurate record can increase the hospital's exposure to liability by destroying the entire record's credibility. In a 1974 Kansas case, the court found that one discrepancy between the medical record and what actually happened to the patient could justify a jury finding that the record could also be erroneous in other parts and be considered generally invalid.[19]

Complete records include observations that the patient's condition has not changed, as well as observations of change. If there is no notation of an observation, many courts permit juries to infer that no observation was made. In 1974, the Illinois Supreme Court decided a case involving a patient admitted with a broken leg.[20] The leg suffered irreversible ischemia while in traction and required amputation. The physician had ordered the nurse to observe the patient's toes, and the medical record indicated hourly observations during the first day of hospitalization. No observations were documented during the seven hours prior to finding the foot cold and without sensation. Though the nurse might have observed the foot during that period, the jury was permitted to infer from the lack of documentation that no observations were made, indicating a breach of the nurse's duty. The hospital, as the nurse's employer, could be liable for resulting injuries.

Failure to document is often also used as an additional offense when providers are charged with other offenses. In 1997, a New York court upheld revocation of a physician's license for a sexual relationship, improper prescribing, and failure to maintain records.[21]

In 1997, a New Jersey court ruled that when errors in records as to time and cause of injury resulted in a low settlement with the person responsible for the injuries, the physician group responsible for the record errors could be sued.[22]

Complete records can often protect hospital and staff. A Kentucky hospital was found not liable for a patient death approximately thirteen hours after surgery because the medical record included documentation of proper periodic nursing observation, contacts with the physician concerning patient management, and compliance with physician directions.[23] Compliance with physician directions does not provide protection when the directions are clearly improper. When the directions are within the range of acceptable professional practice, properly documented compliance provides substantial liability protection.

Medical record entries should usually be made when treatment is given or observations are made. Entries made several days or weeks later have less credibility than those made during or immediately after the patient's hospitalization. Medicare conditions of participation require completion of hospital records within thirty days following patient discharge.[24] TJC's accreditation standards require medical staff regulations to specify a time limit for completion of the record that cannot exceed thirty days after discharge.[25] Persistent failure to conform to this medical staff rule is a basis for suspension of the staff member.[26]

A West Virginia court ruled in favor of a hospital in a case in which a director of social services ordered social workers to review patient charts and complete missing information in master treatment plans for an upcoming accreditation survey. One social worker refused, claiming that it was illegal and then resigned under pressure. The court ruled that completing the plans based on information in the charts was not unethical altering of records.[27]

Medical records should be legible. This does not mean that the patient or another nonhealthcare professional must be able to read the records, but it does mean that other healthcare professionals should be able to read the entries. Otherwise, there is a risk of communication errors that defeat the purpose of the record. Medicare/Medicaid and TJC have long required legible records.[28] In addition, illegible records will not satisfy the other uses of medical records. In 1996, a federal appellate court remanded a disability case because "nontrivial" parts of the medical record were illegible.[29] In 1997, another federal appellate court reversed a judgment in favor of a life insurance company because the only evidence that might support the company was an illegible page of the medical record.[30] In 1999, a physician and pharmacist were found liable for the death of a patient when an illegible prescription was misread.[31] There has been increased public and regulatory attention on legibility.[32] Florida mandated legibility of prescriptions effective July 1, 2003, without specifying penalties, leaving it to the medical licensing board to enforce.[33] In 2003, an Alabama physician lost his license in part for the inability of others to read his prescriptions.[34]

In some circumstances, it is appropriate to use aliases in the place of the names of patients for security or special privacy reasons. This is generally not considered to make the record inaccurate.[35] For example, hospitals that care for high-profile prisoners sometimes give them other names so that persons who seek to help them escape cannot locate them. This is also sometimes done for patients who are celebrities or are under threat from spouses or others. However, there is generally no right to have an alias used.

3.3 How Should Corrections and Alterations in Records Be Handled?

Medical record corrections should be made only by proper methods. Improper alterations reduce record credibility, exposing the hospital to increased liability risk.

Medical record errors can be (1) minor errors in transcription, spelling, and the like or (2) more significant errors involving test data, orders, omitted progress notes, and similar substantive entries. Persons authorized to make record entries may correct minor errors in their own entries soon after the original entry. Hospital policies generally limit who may correct substantive errors and errors discovered at a later date. Those who might have been misled by the error should be notified of changes.

Corrections should be made by placing a single line through the incorrect entry, entering the correct information, initialing or signing the correction, and entering the time and date of the correction. Erasing or obliterating errors can lead jurors to suspect the original entry.

After a claim has been made, changes should not be made without first consulting defense counsel. After several New York physicians won a malpractice suit, it was discovered that a page of the medical record had been replaced before the suit, so the court ordered a new trial.[36] A Maryland court ruled that a malpractice insurer could cancel a physician's coverage for alteration of patient records.[37]

Altering or falsifying a medical record to obtain reimbursement wrongfully is a crime.[38] In some states, a practitioner who improperly alters a medical record is subject to license revocation or other discipline for unprofessional conduct.[39] In some states, improper alteration of a medical record is a crime regardless of the purpose. In 1998, a Virginia appellate court affirmed the conviction of a physician for forging a cardiac stress test record by altering the date. The forgery was used to obtain authorization for coverage of a liver transplant. The physician could be convicted even though the insurer was never billed for the transplant. His medical license was automatically suspended for the conviction, but later reinstated.[40]

Some patients request modification of medical records. Because records are evidence of what occurred and were relied on in making patient care decisions, hospitals should usually not modify records except to update patient name changes. If a patient disagrees with an entry, some hospitals permit amendments in the same manner as corrections of substantive errors if the physician concurs in the amendment. Such an amendment should note the patient's request as a means of explaining the change if it is questioned later. Instead of changing original entries, some hospitals permit patients to add letters to the record. Staff concurrence, if any, can be noted on the letter. Occasionally, courts will order record modifications, especially for records of involuntary evaluation or treatment for mental illness.[41]

3.4 How Long Should Records Be Retained, and How Should They Be Destroyed?

RECORD RETENTION. Because healthcare records are maintained primarily for patient care purposes, decisions concerning record retention periods should be based on sound institutional and medical practice, as well as on applicable regulations. Some states specify minimum retention periods for some or all records. Medicare requires records to be kept for at least five years.[42] Medicare providers must include in contracts with subcontractors a provision requiring the subcontractor to retain records for at least four years after services are provided and to permit the Department of Health and Human Services (HHS) to inspect them.[43] Several state regulations provide that records be kept permanently, but some require retention for the period in which suits may be filed. Some states provide that records cannot be destroyed without state agency approval.

Where there are no controlling regulations, any retention beyond the time needed for medical and administrative purposes should be determined by institutional administration with advice of legal counsel. In institutions where extensive medical research is conducted, a longer retention period may be appropriate to facilitate retrospective studies.

The importance of retaining records until the time has passed for lawsuits is illustrated by a 1984 Florida appellate court decision.[44] The anesthesia records concerning a patient were lost, so the proof necessary to sue the physician was not available. The court ruled that the hospital could be sued for negligently maintaining its records and that the hospital could avoid liability only by showing that the treatment recorded in the missing records was performed nonnegligently, which would be difficult to do without the records.

An independent tort of spoliation of evidence has been recognized by some jurisdictions.[45] Some jurisdictions have limited its applicability.[46] Other jurisdictions have rejected the independent tort.[47]

Sometimes records are lost due to catastrophe such as fire. One federal court permitted the use in a trial of noncontemporaneous medical records created long after the contemporaneous Veterans Administration (VA) hospital records were destroyed in a fire.[48]

RECORD DESTRUCTION. The issue of record destruction arises when the retention period has passed or when a patient requests destruction.

Some state hospital licensing regulations specify the methods for destroying records. The method should protect confidentiality by complete destruction. When required, certificates of destruction should be retained permanently as evidence of record disposal. Some states require creation of a permanent abstract prior to destruction.

Some patients request premature destruction. Some states forbid destruction on an individual basis.[49] In states without specific statutes, it is still prudent not to destroy individual records unless ordered to do so by a court. Courts have generally refused to order destruction. For example, in 1978, the highest court of New York ruled that records could be ordered sealed, but not destroyed.[50] One exception is a 1978 case in which the Pennsylvania Supreme Court ordered destruction of records of the illegal hospitalization of a mental patient.[51]

4 What Are the Laws Concerning Privacy of Healthcare Information?

On April 14, 2003, the laws concerning privacy of healthcare information in the United States were fundamentally changed when the federal privacy regulations under the Health Insurance Portability and Accountability Act (HIPAA) took effect. Any state laws that provide less protection are superseded. State laws that provided more protection remain in effect.

This section addresses the following:

- 4.1. What are the fundamentals of the HIPAA privacy regulations?

- 4.2. What state privacy-related laws remain in effect?

- 4.3. What other federal privacy laws are still applicable?

4.1 What Are the Fundamentals of the HIPAA Privacy Regulations?

The Health Insurance Portability and Accountability Act mandated that HHS issue regulations for the privacy of individually identifiable health information.[52] The privacy rules were initially published in December 2000[53] and then substantially amended in August 2002.[54] The privacy rules took effect April 14, 2003. Courts have rejected challenges to the initial rules and the amended rules.[55] See Figure 1.

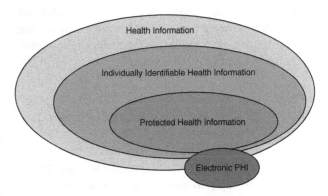

Figure 1 Health Information Rings

HIPAA's Privacy Rule provides that a "Covered Entity" may not use or disclose an individual's "Protected Health Information" unless either the disclosure is permitted under the Privacy Rule or the covered entity has obtained the individual's authorization.[56]

COVERED ENTITIES. The HIPAA privacy rules apply to covered entities.[57] Most healthcare providers, health plans, and healthcare clearinghouses are considered covered entities.

Healthcare providers for whom no health information is transmitted electronically are excluded, but this exception is illusory because it is virtually impossible to provide treatment or bill without electronic transmission of health information, especially because Medicare requires electronic submission of bills.

Initially, HIPAA required covered entities to enter into Business Associate agreements with Business Associates, requiring them to comply with certain privacy requirements.

In 2009, HIPAA was amended to add that "Business Associates" must comply with the Privacy Rule as covered entities do. Business Associates are persons or organizations that (1) perform functions or activities on behalf of a covered entity or (2) provide services to a covered entity that involve the use or disclosure of individually identifiable health information.[58] The types of business associate services that are covered include: legal, actuarial, accounting, consulting, data aggregation, management, administrative, accreditation, and financial services.[59]

PROTECTED HEALTH INFORMATION. The HIPAA privacy rules apply to confidential patient information, which is called protected health information, or PHI, in the rules.[60] PHI includes virtually all individually identifiable health information, which is defined to include any health information, including demographic information collected from the individual, that:

(1) Is created or received by a healthcare provider, health plan, employer, or healthcare clearinghouse; and

(2) Relates to the past, present, or future physical or mental health or condition of an individual; the provision of health care to an individual; or the past, present, or future payment for the provision of health care to an individual; and

(i) That identifies the individual; or

(ii) With respect to which there is a reasonable basis to believe the information can be used to identify the individual.[60]

When there is no reasonable basis to believe the information can be used to identify the individual, the PHI and the HIPAA rules do not apply. The HIPAA privacy rules apply to PHI in all formats—written, spoken, or electronic.

NOTICE OF PRIVACY PRACTICES. HIPAA requires that upon initial presentation to a healthcare provider, all patients must be given a notice of privacy practices.[61] A record must be kept of giving this notice. Generally, the patient or patient's representative will be asked to sign an acknowledgment.

SAFEGUARDS. HIPAA requires covered entities to take steps to safeguard PHI.[62] They must train their workforces to take common sense steps so that unauthorized persons do not come into contact with PHI. This ranges from not leaving medical records where they can be seen by the public to not talking about patients in cafeterias and elevators, and adopting security standards for providers' computers and handheld devices.

PATIENT AUTHORIZATION. HIPAA permits many internal uses and external disclosures of PHI without patient authorization. In general, uses and disclosures for treatment, payment, or healthcare operations are permitted without authorization.[63] Many disclosures that are required to safeguard the public, such as child abuse reporting, are also permitted.[64] These and other permitted uses and disclosures are discussed in sections 5 and 6.

Other uses and disclosures generally require authorization from the patient or the patient's representative. There are a few uses, such as listing in a facility directory, where all that is required is that the patient be given an opportunity to object.[65]

It is important for providers to understand which activities can be conducted without patient authorization and which activities require patient authorization.

MINIMUM NECESSARY. Most of the permitted uses and disclosures of PHI are subject to the minimum necessary rule, which requires that uses or disclosures be limited to the minimum necessary information for the permitted purpose.[66]

ALTERNATIVE COMMUNICATIONS. HIPAA requires that patients may request that healthcare providers contact them in a certain way, such as to leave a message on voice mail. Reasonable requests should usually be accommodated.[67]

ACCESS TO RECORDS. HIPAA requires that patients generally may look at their medical and billing records and make copies.[68]

CHANGES TO RECORDS. HIPAA requires that patients may ask for their medical or billing records to be changed, but patients do not have a right to compel changes.[69]

TRACKING OF DISCLOSURES. HIPAA requires that covered entities must maintain a record of some types of disclosures. With a few exceptions, patients have the right to see this list and get a copy of it.[70]

RESTRICTIONS ON USE. HIPAA requires that patients may request restrictions on the use of their patient information, but covered entities are not required to agree to such restrictions.[71] When they do agree, they must comply with their agreements.[72]

ADMINISTRATIVE STEPS. Covered entities are required to have a designated privacy officer, create policies and procedures, train workers, accept privacy complaints, and take corrective steps when there are violations.[73]

MARKETING AND FUNDRAISING. The HIPAA privacy rules generally prohibit using PHI for marketing of healthcare services or fundraising, unless authorization is obtained from the patient or patient's representative.[74]

The HHS Office for Civil Rights (OCR) enforces the privacy rules.

According to the HHS Office for Civil Rights website, the Privacy Rule compliance issues investigated most are: (1) Impermissible uses and disclosures of protected health information; (2) Lack of safeguards of protected health information; (3) Lack of patient access to their protected health information; (4) Uses or disclosures of more than the Minimum Necessary protected health information; and (5) Complaints to the covered entity. The types of covered entities that have most commonly been required to take corrective action to achieve compliance with the Privacy Rule are, in order of frequency: (1) Private Practices; (2) General Hospitals; (3) Outpatient Facilities; (4) Health Plans (group health plans and health insurance issuers); and (5) Pharmacies.

Unlike many other HHS enforcement efforts, the OCR has kept a low profile in its enforcement, focusing its efforts on promoting compliance rather than punishment. Until July 2004, there were no publicized impositions of penalties, although there were reports that unidentified cases had been referred to the Department of Justice for possible prosecution.[76] In August 2004, the first conviction was announced. A Washington healthcare worker pled guilty to having used information from a patient's medical records to obtain credit cards in the patient's name.[77] The facility cooperated in the investigation and was not charged. In June 2005, the U.S. Department of Justice announced that the criminal penalties of HIPAA generally do not apply to individual employees of providers; instead, they apply to insurers, physicians, hospitals, and other providers.[78] In February 2011, the OCR issued the first Civil Monetary Penalty for a violation of the HIPAA privacy rule. Cignet Health of Prince George's County, Maryland ("Cignet"), was fined $4.3 million for denying patients access to their medical records. Specifically, Cignet was fined $1.3 million for failing to give 41 patients access to their medical records between September 2008 and October 2009, and $3 million for failing to cooperate with the OCR investigation.

There is no private cause of action for enforcement of the HIPAA privacy rules.[79] This means that patients and their representatives cannot sue providers seeking payment for violation of HIPAA privacy rules. Patients and their representatives must rely on remedies under other laws. Enforcement of the HIPAA privacy rules is left to the OCR.

4.2 What State Privacy-Related Laws Remain in Effect?

HIPAA preempts any state laws that provide less protection, but any state law that provides as great or greater protections than HIPAA remains in effect.[80] Thus, state laws that restrict access to certain information at least as strictly as HIPAA remain in effect.

The general state laws concerning confidentiality of healthcare information also remain important. Because there is no private cause of action under the HIPAA privacy rules, state laws remain as the basis for some private causes of action. States can still enforce individual and institutional licensing rules and criminal laws[81] that generally require confidentiality.

The HIPAA privacy rules permit attorneys to issue subpoenas of PHI without a court order when certain procedural steps are followed. Some states, such as Wisconsin, do not permit this practice, requiring a court order when discovery of PHI is sought without a written authorization of the patient.

The HIPAA privacy rules also recognize the broad authority of courts to order release of PHI. Most states have placed significantly more limitations on the scope of courts to order release of PHI than has the federal government. These state laws continue to be constraints on the judiciary, at least in the cases where state law must be followed. The physician-patient privilege is one of the most important constraints on judicial disclosure of PHI.

MENTAL HEALTH. Many states have statutes that limit access to and disclosure of mental health information. In 1998, an Illinois appellate court ruled that it was a violation of the state confidentiality statute to voluntarily disclose mental health records to a physician appointed by a court to examine a patient for involuntary commitment.[82] In 1996, a federal appellate court applied the state mental health records law to issue a writ of mandamus commanding a lower court not to require a hospital to produce the records of two male patients who had allegedly raped the plaintiff.[83]

HIV/AIDS. Many states have statutes that specify when an HIV test result or a diagnosis of AIDS can be disclosed.[84] These statutes are often strictly interpreted.

A California physician was sued for writing a patient's HIV status in a medical record without the written consent required by state law, even though the patient had given verbal consent. The physician settled the suit.[85] A New York physician was found to have violated the law by disclosing a positive HIV test to an out-of-state workers' compensation board, where the authorization from the patient did not satisfy the statutory requirements.[86] Placing a red sticker on the possessions of a HIV-positive inmate and segregating her improperly disclosed her HIV status to persons who were not authorized to know.[87] In 2004, a District of Columbia court ruled that the law did not prohibit a physician from discussing the case of an HIV-positive patient with another physician in the same office.[88]

However, a Pennsylvania court permitted a hospital to make limited disclosure of a resident physician's HIV-positive status, including disclosure to patients without naming the resident.[89]

A North Carolina court upheld revocation of the clinical privileges of a physician for not complying with a hospital policy that required disclosure to the hospital of any inpatient who was HIV-positive.[90]

In some states, these laws require reporting of HIV/AIDS and disclosure to partners and others.[91]

COMMON LAW. The common law usually does not provide any protection from disclosure in testimonial contexts (e.g., trials, court hearings, subpoenas). Courts generally refuse to impose liability for testimonial disclosures.[92] Physicians and hospitals are usually not obligated to risk contempt of court to protect confidences (except for substance abuse records), although they might choose to do so.

In nontestimonial contexts, courts have found limitations on permissible disclosure based on the implied promise of confidentiality in the physician-patient relationship, violation of the right of privacy, and violation of professional licensing standards.[93] For example, a New York court permanently enjoined a psychoanalyst from circulating a book that included detailed information concerning a patient.[94] The patient was identifiable to close friends despite the psychoanalyst's efforts to disguise her identity. The court ruled that the book violated the implied covenant of confidentiality and the right of privacy. The Oregon Supreme Court held that a physician could be liable for revealing his patient's identity to the patient's natural child, who had been adopted.[95] The court ruled that while it was not a violation of the patient's right of privacy, it was a breach of the physician's professional duty to maintain the patient's confidentiality.

Courts have ruled in favor of healthcare providers in cases where disclosure was intended to prevent the spread of contagious disease or the patient was in a dangerous mental state.[96] As discussed in the section on the common law duty to disclose information, there could be liability in some circumstances for failing to disclose a contagious disease or dangerous mental state. Disclosures to the patient's employer or insurance company have resulted in several lawsuits.[97] The Alabama Supreme Court ruled that disclosures to an employer without authorization violated the implied promise of confidentiality and could result in liability.[98] The employer who induces the disclosure can also be liable.[99] However, a New York court ruled that when a patient authorized incomplete disclosure to his employer that the physician was not liable for giving a complete disclosure.[100] It is questionable whether other courts would rule this way, so the prudent practice is to refuse to release any information when only a misleading partial release is authorized.

Lawsuits for disclosures of confidential informatio have also been based on defamation. In most cases involving physicians, courts have found a qualified privilege to make the specific disclosures.[101] The few cases of liability have involved disclosure of a misdiagnosed embarrassing condition (such as venereal disease) that the patient did not actually have in a manner that demonstrated malice, defeating the qualified privilege.[102]

Misuse of confidential information without disclosure can also lead to sanctions. In 1991, a New York psychiatrist pled guilty to securities fraud for trading in stocks based on inside information received from a patient.[103]

Courts have disagreed on whether claims concerning release of information are subject to state medical malpractice claims procedures.[104]

PHYSICIAN-PATIENT PRIVILEGE. The physician-patient privilege is the rule that a physician is not permitted to testify as a witness concerning certain information gained in the physician-patient relationship. There was no physician-patient privilege from testimonial disclosure under the English common law. Nearly all U.S. courts also have adopted this position, so with few exceptions, the privilege exists only in states that have enacted privilege statutes. One exception is Alaska, which established a common law psychotherapist-patient privilege for criminal cases.[105] Federal courts must apply state privileges in lawsuits concerning state law, but state privileges do not apply in most federal lawsuits concerning federal law.[106]

Approximately two thirds of the states have enacted a statutory physician-patient privilege. Privilege statutes address only situations in which the physician is being compelled to testify, such as in a deposition, administrative hearing, or trial or to release subpoenaed records. There is a widespread misperception that privilege statutes apply to other disclosures, but in most states, this is not true.[107] The duty to maintain confidentiality outside of testimonial contexts is grounded on other statutes and legal principles. Thus, privilege statutes are usually of concern only when providers are responding to legal compulsion.

The privilege applies only when a bona fide physician-patient relationship exists. The privilege usually does not apply to court-ordered examinations or other examinations solely for the benefit of third parties, such as insurance companies.

The scope of the privilege varies. Pennsylvania limits the privilege to communications that tend to blacken the character of the patient,[108] while Kansas extends the privilege to all communications and observations.[109] Michigan limits the privilege to physicians,[110] while New York extends the privilege to dentists and nurses.[111] When a nurse is present during a confidential communication between a physician and a patient, some states extend the privilege to the nurse, while other states rule that the communication is no longer privileged for the physician. Generally, the privilege extends to otherwise privileged information recorded in the hospital record.[112] However, information that is required to be reported to public authorities has generally been held not to be privileged unless the public authorities are also privileged not to disclose it.

Even when privileges otherwise apply, most state statutes include numerous exemptions from the privilege.[113] They vary between states.

Psychotherapist-Patient Privilege. In many states, a separate statute establishes a psychotherapist-patient privilege. The definition of a psychotherapist varies. The Georgia Supreme Court ruled that the state psychiatrist-patient privilege applied to nonpsychiatrists who devoted a substantial part of their time to mental diseases.[114]

In 1996, the U.S. Supreme Court recognized a federal psychotherapist-patient privilege.[115] The Supreme Court left open the possibility that a dangerous patient exception might develop, but federal appellate courts have refused to create such an exception.[116] In 2000, a federal appellate court ruled that parties waive the privilege when they place their medical condition in issue.[117]

Because most third-party payers require waiver of the privilege before providing payment, some psychotherapists make other arrangements with patients for payment to protect confidentiality.[118]

Waiver. The patient may waive the privilege, permitting the physician to testify. The privilege can be waived by contract. Insurance applications and policies often include waivers. Other actions can constitute implied waiver. Introducing evidence of medical details or failing to object to physician testimony generally waives the privilege.[119] Authorization of disclosure outside the testimonial context usually does not waive the privilege.[120] Thus, the patient generally may authorize other persons to have access to medical records outside of court and still successfully object to having them introduced into evidence unless other actions have waived the privilege. In a few states, authorization of any disclosure to opposing parties waives the privilege.[121] One federal appellate court has ruled that any disclosure to a third party waives the federal psychotherapist-patient privilege.[122]

Making a claim based on emotional distress or other mental condition usually waives the psychotherapist-patient privilege.[123] In some states, if the mental claim is dropped from the suit, the privilege is restored.[124]

Waiver of the privilege usually permits only formal discovery and testimony, not informal interviews. Express patient consent is generally required before informal interviews are permitted.[125] Other courts have permitted informal interviews based on waiver of the privilege.[126] However, in some states, it may be breach of the physician's duty to the patient to engage in informal interviews.[127] Most providers limit disclosures to formal channels unless express patient consent is obtained. One federal trial court has ruled that the HIPAA privacy rules impose this requirement of express consent to informal interviews.[128]

4.3 What Other Federal Privacy Laws Are Still Applicable?

The HIPAA privacy rules are not the only federal privacy laws applicable to healthcare information. For example, the federal substance abuse confidentiality rules remain in effect.

SUBSTANCE ABUSE. Special federal rules deal with confidentiality of information concerning patients treated or referred for treatment for alcoholism or drug abuse.[129] The rules apply to any specialized program for substance abuse in any facility receiving federal funds for any purpose, including Medicare or Medicaid reimbursement. Since 1994, the rules have not applied to treatment outside of specialized programs, so they do not apply to most emergency room treatments.[130]

The regulations preempt any state law that purports to authorize disclosures contrary to the regulations, but states are permitted to impose tighter confidentiality requirements. The rules apply to any disclosure, even acknowledgment of the patient's presence in the facility. Information may be released with the patient's consent if the consent is in writing and contains all the elements required by the federal rules.

A court order, including a subpoena, does not permit release of information unless the requirements of the regulations have all been met.[131] The regulations require a court hearing and a court finding that the purpose for which the order is sought is more important than the purpose for which Congress mandated confidentiality. The regulations have been interpreted to permit hospitals to tell the court why they cannot comply with the order

until after a hearing. After a hearing, courts have ordered disclosures to assist probation revocation and child abuse proceedings,[132] to assist an Internal Revenue Service investigation of a surgeon,[133] and other situations.[134] Courts have declined to order disclosure when the information was sought to challenge the credibility of witnesses, assist in determining the rehabilitation potential of a convicted person for purposes of sentencing, or assist in a drug possession investigation.[135]

Child abuse reports may be made under state law without patient consent or a court order, but release of records to child abuse agencies requires consent or an order.

Federal courts have ruled that the federal substance abuse rules do not create a private cause of action for violations, so that only the federal government can sue for violations.[136]

FAMILY EDUCATIONAL RIGHTS AND PRIVACY ACT (FERPA). Strict federal rules preclude universities from sharing information about students with their parents or others without the students' consent.[137] This has created controversial situations where schools have not been able to involve parents in dealing with suicidal behaviors.[138] The HIPAA privacy rules do not apply to records that are subject to FERPA.[139]

FAIR AND ACCURATE CREDIT TRANSACTIONS ACT. There are federal restrictions on the use of medical information in credit reports.[140]

PRIVACY ACT. The Privacy Act[141] prohibits disclosures of records contained in a system of records maintained by a federal agency (or its contractors) without the written request or consent of the individual to whom the record pertains, subject to various statutory exceptions.

In some cases, the Privacy Act may prohibit some disclosures permitted by the HIPAA privacy rules. The preamble to the December 2000 HIPAA privacy rules indicates that the HIPAA privacy rules may prohibit some disclosures permitted by the Privacy Act and in those cases the HIPAA privacy rules must be followed.

5 What Are the Laws Concerning Use of Healthcare Information?

The HIPAA privacy rules permit broad uses of PHI for treatment, payment, and healthcare operations without patient authorization. This is subject to the requirement that the covered entity has privacy policies, workforce members are trained on the requirements, and contractors who have access to the information have a business associate agreement with the covered entity addressing the requirements.

These uses are generally subject to the minimum necessary standards mentioned in section   4.1.

State law has long recognized that providers must be able to use PHI, so the HIPAA privacy rules are consistent with the law of most states.

TREATMENT. Those who are involved in patient care must have timely access to records to fulfill the patient care functions of the records. Records must be readily accessible for present and future patient care. There will always be some risk of occasional unauthorized access by others.

In the past, some courts have tried to draw a distinction between diagnosis and treatment. HIPAA expressly rejects this distinction; treatment is defined to include "the provision, coordination, or management of health care and related services by one or more health care providers" and health care is defined to include diagnosis.[142]

HIPAA includes within the definition of permitted treatment uses the exchange of information among providers for consultation, referrals, and other treatment purposes. It is not unusual for a provider to need to know about the prior or concurrent treatment from other providers.

PAYMENT. Providers must be able to use healthcare information to process claims for payment. Payers have a legitimate need for data to justify their payments, and providers must be able to provide that data. State laws also recognize this.[143] HIPAA broadly defines what is in the scope of payment.[144]

HEALTHCARE OPERATIONS. HIPAA broadly defines the scope of healthcare operations.[145] Medical records are also business records. Many staff members must have access to medical records to operate the healthcare organization. An organization has authority to permit internal access by professional, technical, and administrative personnel who need access.

Under prior law, these administrative uses were so widely understood that they were seldom addressed in reported court decisions. The few cases were decided in favor of administrative access. In 1965, the highest court of New York authorized a trustee to examine medical records of patients involved in a controversial research project.[146] In

Examples of tasks which may require access to medical records include: • Auditing • Filing • Replying to inquiries • Quality improvement • Risk management • Defending potential litigation

1975, a Missouri court upheld the authority of hospitals to review records for quality assurance purposes.[147] In 1979, a Canadian court ruled that the hospital's insurers and lawyers may have access to prepare to deal with patient claims.[148] However, in 1999, the Ohio Supreme Court ruled that a hospital could not share its records with a law firm that was hired to screen medical records to locate patients who could seek government payments.[149] Other courts have not placed this limit on the ability of hospitals to use agents. Some plaintiffs' attorneys have attempted to bar hospital attorneys from communicating with physicians and hospital employees involved in the case without the presence of the plaintiffs' attorneys. Courts have generally rejected these attempts.[150]

RESEARCH. Prior to the HIPAA privacy rules, healthcare providers generally could use their own records to conduct medical research without patient consent. Federal human subject regulations and many state laws expressly authorized this practice. Federal human subject regulations exempted some research involving only records from review processes or made the research eligible for expedited review.[151] Important medical discoveries have been made through researching medical records.[152]

The HIPAA privacy rules essentially eliminated the exemption from review. An institutional review board or privacy board must review all records research, and patient authorization must be obtained unless an institutional review board or privacy board grants a waiver of authorization.[153]

6 What Are the Laws Concerning Disclosure of Healthcare Information?

Courts generally adhere to the doctrine of stare decisis, which is frequently described as "following precedent." This section discusses the circumstances in which healthcare information can or must be disclosed outside of the covered entity and those working for the covered entity.

The following questions are addressed:

- 6.1. When can the patient or representative authorize disclosure of PHI?
- 6.2. When and how can disclosure be compelled in legal proceedings?
- 6.3. When are providers required or authorized to report PHI to legal authorities and others?
- 6.4. When may providers disclose PHI in response to inquiries from legal authorities?
- 6.5. When may providers disclose PHI in response to inquiries from others?

6.1 When Can the Patient or Representative Authorize Disclosure of PHI?

With rare exceptions, the patient (or representative of an incapacitated patient) may authorize release of PHI to themselves or others.

AUTHORIZATION BY PATIENT. Competent patients can generally authorize access to themselves and others. The HIPAA privacy regulations recognize this right, while permitting withholding of information in limited circumstances if specified procedures are followed.[154]

The right of access by the patient has been widely recognized prior to HIPAA either through statutes or court decisions.[155] In 1986, a Pennsylvania court found that denial of access could be intentional infliction of emotional distress.[156] In 1990, the Maryland high court ruled that a hospital could be assessed punitive damages for failing to provide requested medical records within a reasonable time.[157]

In 1994, a Florida appellate court ruled that a healthcare provider could require that the patient's signature on a release form be notarized.[158] This case should not be interpreted to suggest that notarization is necessary. However, it is clear that courts will accept identity checks that are appropriate to the situation.

Providers generally cannot condition release of records on prior arrangements for payment for the documented care. In 1997, a California appellate court ruled that a provider could not require the patient to sign a lien before releasing records.[159]

The right to authorize others to have access has also been widely recognized prior to HIPAA.[160]

HIPAA generally permits disclosures to family members, relatives, and close friends who are involved in the patient's care, unless the patient objects.[161] In essence, there is implied authorization to keep those involved in the patient's care informed, unless the patient objects or other law prohibits the disclosure. The federal substance abuse confidentiality rules discussed in section 4.3 restrict disclosures related to substance abuse treatment.

Release of psychiatric information is subject to special restrictions in some states. In 1982, a New York court stated that a spouse should not be given psychiatric information, even when there is no estrangement, unless (1) the patient authorizes disclosure or (2) a danger to the patient, spouse, or another person can be reduced by disclosure.[162] Some states authorize disclosure of psychiatric information to spouses and others in additional circumstances.[163]

Providers can refuse to release records until presented with a release form that complies with their reasonable policies. A Missouri court upheld a hospital's refusal to release records to an attorney who presented a form with an altered date.[164]

When providers agree to release information, they may be liable for failing to do so. In 1999, a federal appellate court ruled that a former patient could sue a psychiatric facility, when a staff member failed to fulfill a promise to inform the patient's employer that the employee was unable to come to work.[165]

EXCEPTIONS. The HIPAA privacy rules recognize that there are some circumstances where release of the information to the patient can endanger the life or physical safety of the patient and permit withholding information in such cases subject to a right to have the decision reviewed.[166] Courts had previously recognized some exceptions to the general rule in favor of access. Courts have generally insisted that medically contraindicated information be made available to the patient's representative, who is frequently an outside professional acting on behalf of the patient. For example, in 1979, a federal appellate court addressed the withholding of information from patients preparing for hearings challenging their transfer to a lower level of care.[167] The court ruled that it was not enough for the state to offer to release information to a representative when the patient did not have a representative. The state was permitted to withhold medically contraindicated information from patients only when they had representatives, provided by the state if necessary.

Mental health information is treated differently in some circumstances. In 1995, the Utah Supreme Court ruled that a mental health clinic could assert a privilege not to disclose its records even after the patient executed a release document.[168] In a 1983 case, a New York mental hospital attempted to enforce its policy of releasing records only to physicians.[169] The court ruled that the records could be protected from disclosure only if the hospital proved release would cause detriment (1) to the patient, (2) to involved third parties, or (3) to an important hospital program. Because none of these was proved, the court ordered disclosure to the persons authorized by the patient. In 1997, a federal court ruled that a Florida statute denying persons with mental conditions access to obtain their medical records after discharge discriminated against persons with mental disabilities, violating the Americans with Disabilities Act.[170]

AUTHORIZATION BY THE PATIENT'S REPRESENTATIVE. When authorization is required and the patient is unable to authorize access because of incapacity, minority, or death, someone other than the patient must authorize access. The HIPAA privacy rules state that a personal representative of the patient has the same rights as the patient and specifies how to determine who may be a personal representative.[171]

Mentally Incapacitated Patients. The HIPAA privacy rules generally look to state law to identify the personal representative. Anyone that state law permits to make medical decisions is a personal representative. Some courts have suppressed family confidences and information that could upset the patient severely.[172] Similarly, the HIPAA privacy rules permit withholding information that is reasonably likely to cause substantial harm.[173]

In 2004, a New York court ruled that under the HIPAA privacy rules an agent under an activated healthcare proxy was entitled to access.[174]

When the mental incapacity is temporary and the release of the information can reasonably wait, it usually is appropriate to wait for the patient's authorization.

MINORS. The HIPAA privacy rules generally look to state law to determine when a parent or other individual who has assumed parental rights, duties, and obligations is the personal representative and may authorize disclosure of PHI.[175] For most minors, state laws provide for the decision whether to release records to be made by a custodial parent. Access rights of noncustodial parents vary from state to state and can depend on the specific wording of the applicable court order assigning custodial rights.[176]

States vary greatly in the extent to which older minors are allowed to control access of parents and guardians to records.[177] Some state statutes specify that information regarding certain types of treatment, such as treatment for venereal disease and substance abuse, cannot be disclosed without the minor's consent. Some statutes specify that parents must be informed before a minor obtains certain kinds of services.[178]

In some states, when minors may legally consent to their own care, parents do not have a right to information concerning the care. If the minor fails to make other arrangements to pay for the care and relies on the parents to pay, the parents can be entitled to more information.

Providers generally can release information concerning immature minors to custodial parents without substantial risk of liability unless state statutes expressly prohibit release. When a mature minor wishes information withheld from parents, the provider must make a professional judgment concerning information release to the parents except in the few circumstances where the law is settled, such as when a constitutional statute requires or forbids notification. Disclosure is generally permitted when there is likelihood of harm (such as contagious disease) to the minor or others and avoidance of that harm requires parental involvement.

STATE STATUTES SHOULD BE FOLLOWED. A Georgia court ruled that a father could sue a psychiatrist for releasing his minor daughter's mental health records to his former wife's attorney for use in custody litigation.[179] The daughter had requested the release and had ratified it after becoming an adult, but the release did not comply with the state statute.

DECEASED PATIENTS. The HIPAA privacy rules apply after the death of the patient.[180] The executor, administrator, or other person authorized to act on behalf of the deceased individual or estate may act as the personal representative.[181] Disclosures can be made without authorization for some law enforcement purposes, disposal of the body, or cadaveric organ donation.[182]

If there is an executor or administrator of the estate, required authorizations should usually be sought from that person.[183] If there is no executor or administrator, in most states authorization should be obtained from the next of kin, such as a surviving spouse[184] or a child.[185] Authorizations signed by the patient before death may still apply.[186]

The Wisconsin Supreme Court ruled that a hospital could insist that the person signing an authorization for release of the records of a deceased person state the authority of the person signing.[187]

6.2 When and How Can Disclosure Be Compelled in Legal Proceedings?

Even if the patient or representative opposes information release, healthcare providers can be compelled by law to disclose information in legal proceedings through subpoenas and other procedures to discover evidence.

In lawsuits and administrative proceedings, the parties are authorized by law to demand relevant unprivileged information in the control of others. Lawyers call this the discovery process.

SUBPOENAS AND OTHER DISCOVERY ORDERS. The most frequent discovery demand is called a subpoena. A subpoena is a request for production of documents, or a request for an individual to appear in court or other legal proceeding. In federal courts and in most states, demands to parties are generally called notices of deposition or notices to produce, while actual subpoenas are used only for persons who are not parties to the suit. Notices and subpoenas have essentially the same effect, so what is said about subpoenas in the rest of this chapter also applies to notices. When the demands are ignored, a court can order compliance, and further noncompliance can be punished as contempt of court. Contempt of court is a court order which, in the context of a court trial or hearing, declares a person or organization to have disobeyed or been disrespectful of the court's authority. A judge may hold a litigant "in contempt," and may even impose sanctions, when the judge determines the person has disrupted the court's orderly process.

In some jurisdictions, a subpoena is issued by the court and constitutes a court order. A court order is generally sufficient authorization to release a medical record, unless special protections apply. For example, federal rules require a court order before substance abuse records may be released.

In some jurisdictions where individual attorneys are permitted to issue subpoenas without involvement of a court, noncourt subpoenas are not sufficient authorization to release medical records in some circumstances.[188] In those circumstances, the provider should assert the confidentiality of the records and demand a court order or authorization from the patient or an appropriate representative.[189]

Some states have sought to simplify the discovery process by mandating exchange of records. However, such requirements are not universal. For example, in 1997, the Illinois Supreme Court declared such a law to be an unconstitutional violation of the separation of powers and of privacy rights.[190]

HIPAA REQUIREMENTS. The HIPAA privacy rules permit subpoenas and other court-ordered releases of PHI. However, when a subpoena is issued without a court order, the covered entity must be provided with assurances that there have been reasonable efforts to notify the patient or obtain a protective order.[191]

RESPONSES TO SUBPOENAS AND OTHER DISCOVERY ORDERS. In most situations, the proper response to a valid subpoena or discovery order is compliance. However, prompt legal assistance should be sought because some subpoenas or orders are not valid and others should be resisted.[192] A discovery order should never be ignored. A subpoena is part of a court's legal process and failure to respond is considered contempt of court in most states.

Subpoenas from state courts in other states are usually not valid unless they are given to the person being subpoenaed while that person is in the state of the issuing court. For example, in 1993, a New York appellate court ruled that a New York physician could be sued for releasing information pursuant to a Pennsylvania state subpoena.[193] Courts in some states have authority to issue subpoenas to persons only in a limited area. Most states have a procedure for obtaining a valid subpoena from a local court to require the release of information for a trial in a distant court that does not have the authority to issue a valid subpoena. Some state courts will order a party to sign a document requesting and authorizing release of records, especially out-of-state records, instead of going through the process of obtaining an order where the records are located.[194]

Subpoenas from federal courts in other states are usually valid.

Sometimes challenges to subpoenas are successful. A New Jersey court refused to order a woman or her psychiatrist to answer questions concerning nonfinancial matters in a marriage separation case because the husband had failed to demonstrate relevance or good cause for the order.[195] When judges are not certain whether to order a release, they sometimes will order that the information be presented for court review before ruling.[196]

In some situations, the only way to obtain prompt appellate review of an apparently inappropriate discovery order is to risk being found in contempt of court. In one case a physician challenged a grand jury subpoena of records of sixty-three patients.[197] The trial court found the physician to be in contempt for failing to comply. The Illinois Supreme Court held that he must release the records of the one patient who had waived her physician-patient privilege but reversed the contempt finding on the other sixty-two records. They were protected by the physician-patient privilege in Illinois until a showing of a criminal action relating to the treatment documented in the records was made. In another Illinois case, the appellate court ruled that the trial court had erred in jailing a physician and his attorney for contempt of court concerning a deposition. The applicable statute did not permit more discovery than had been given, and the trial court failed to show any accommodation for the patients scheduled for the physician's care.[198]

Valid subpoenas should never be ignored and should never be challenged except on advice of an attorney, but attorneys should be cautious in giving such advice. A federal court found an attorney to be in contempt and fined the attorney for advising the client to resist a subpoena in a Medicare investigation.[199]

MEDICAL INFORMATION. A subpoena can require that medical records (or copies) be provided to the court or to the other side in the suit. If an individual's physical or mental condition is at issue in the litigation, he or she may also be ordered to submit to a physical or mental examination. During a deposition, a person submits to formal questioning under oath prior to the trial. Deposition testimony may later be used as testimony at trial, if the person questioned is unavailable to testify in person during the trial.

PARTIES. Under the current liberal discovery practices, medical records of parties can nearly always be subpoenaed if the mental or physical condition of the party is relevant. Further, those who provided the health care may be ordered to give depositions.

NONPARTIES. In most circumstances, courts will not permit discovery of information concerning health care of persons who are not parties.[200] Some attorneys have sought such information to establish what happened when similar treatment was given to other patients. Providers have resisted these attempts on the basis that they invade patient privacy, violate the physician-patient privilege discussed in a later section, and are not relevant because of the uniqueness of the condition and reaction of each patient.

The only widely accepted exceptions in which discovery of nonparty records has been permitted have been cases of billing fraud or professional discipline.[201] Some courts have permitted access to medical records of nonparties in malpractice suits but have required all "identifiers" to be deleted.[202] However, other courts have reaffirmed the traditional rule and declined to order access even with identifiers deleted.[203]

PATIENT NAMES. Some attorneys have attempted to bypass the rule against disclosure of nonparty medical records by seeking nonparty patients' names and obtaining their permission to get the records. Providers have resisted these attempts for reasons similar to those for resisting discovery of records. Most courts have not permitted discovery of nonparty patient names. For example, in 2002, the Illinois Supreme Court considered a case where the Department of Professional Regulation subpoenaed the medical records of two individuals who were not parties to the case. The Illinois Supreme Court ruled that merely deleting patient names and other identifying information from patient records before disclosing them violated the physician-patient privilege.[204] In 2004, the Supreme Court of New York held that the discovery of nonparty patient names and addresses violated the physician-patient privilege.[205] Similarly, in 2006, the Superior Court of New Jersey held that information that a patient communicates in confidence to a physician or hospital that is protected from disclosure by the physician-patient privilege includes the patient's name and address.[206]

COMMITTEE REPORTS. Many states have enacted statutes protecting quality improvement and peer review activities and committee reports from discovery or admission into evidence. Peer review is the process by which a committee of physicians examines the work of a peer and determines whether the physician under review has met the accepted standard of medical care. Laws protecting the confidentiality of information discovered during the peer review process are intended to encourage self-regulation by the medical profession through peer review and evaluation. Courts have found these laws constitutional.[207]

Different states have taken different stances with respect to the extent to which the activities and reports of peer review committees should be protected. Some courts have strictly interpreted statutory protections, reducing their effectiveness. For example, in 2009, the Colorado Supreme Court held that Colorado's peer review statute prevented the proceedings of a medical review committee engaged in the process of peer review from being subject to discovery or introduction into evidence in a civil action, but did not bar the disclosure of such information pursuant to the Connecticut Freedom of Information Act.[208] Similarly, a New Jersey court refused to extend the statutory protection for "utilization review committees" to related committees, such as the medical records committee and infection control committee.[209] In 2007, the Florida Supreme Court considered whether Florida's peer review law protected a list generated by a hospital, which included a peer review committee recommendation delineating the privileges given to a member of a hospital staff.[210] The court held that the peer review statute did not exempt the hospital from disclosure of its decision to grant or deny certain practice privileges to a physician.[211] Similarly, the Georgia Supreme Court held that to the extent that there was information in a physician's credentialing files that did not involve a peer review committee's evaluations of his performance of medical procedures, that information was discoverable.[212]

The decision of a West Virginia court is illustrative of the hostility of some courts towards peer review and committee privileges. In that case, the court ruled that judges should not rely on a hospital's assertion of the privilege, but instead should inspect all the documents for which the privilege was claimed and require the hospital to prove that each document was protected by the privilege.[213]

In other jurisdictions, however, courts have interpreted statutory protections more broadly.[214] In 2009, the Alabama Supreme Court, in construing Alabama's peer review statute, stated that the statute protected any document considered by the peer review committee or hospital board in its decision-making process.[215] The Minnesota Supreme Court found that a complications conference report was protected under a statute that protected "the proceedings and records of a review organization."[216] Under some states' laws, the identities of persons involved in peer review are also protected.[217] In 2005, an Ohio appellate court ruled that a hospital did not have to produce a list of peer reviewed documents in order to assert the privilege for them.[218]

Some state laws only protect peer review records from discovery; if they are obtained through other channels they can be used in court.[219] Other laws protect the records from being introduced in lawsuits even if they are obtained outside discovery channels.[220]

Even when the privilege does apply, many state laws permit state licensing agencies to gain access.[221] This can become a significant loophole in the protection of peer review committee information. For example, in 1998, the Kansas Supreme Court permitted private plaintiffs to access and use most of the records the state licensing agency had obtained.[222]

In addition to protections afforded by individual state statutes, federal law also provides some safeguards for information generated in the course of peer review activities. The Health Care Quality Improvement Act (HCQIA) provides immunity from damages to participants in a professional review action if the action meets certain standards and follows certain procedures.[223] HCQIA provides this immunity as an "incentive and protection for physicians engaging in effective professional peer review."[224] In enacting HCQIA, Congress believed that effective peer review, including mandatory reporting to a nationwide database, could alleviate the national problem of "the increasing occurrence of medical malpractice" by "restricting the ability of incompetent physicians to move from State to State without disclosure or discovery of the physician's previous damaging or incompetent performance."[225] However, HCQIA does not provide unqualified immunity to all peer review decisions. In order to ensure that such review is effective and not abused, HCQIA only provides immunity to "professional review actions" based on a physician's "competence or professional conduct,"[226] and it mandates specific standards and procedures that must be followed.[227]

Nevertheless, because the status of committee reports is still an open question in many states, these reports should be carefully written so that, if they must be released, they will not inappropriately increase liability exposure.

PATIENT SAFETY ORGANIZATIONS. Information pertaining to medical errors may also be protected from discovery in litigation if it is reported to an authorized Patient Safety Organization (PSO). In 1999, the Institutes of Medicine published a report entitled "To Err is Human, Building a Safer Health System," detailing the enormous human, financial, and societal impact of preventable medical errors each year.[228] The report called on Congress to establish a network of independent patient safety organizations nationwide. As a response, the federal Patient Safety and Quality Improvement Act was signed into law in 2005.[229]

The federal Patient Safety and Quality Improvement Act creates PSOs to collect, aggregate, and analyze confidential information reported by healthcare providers.

The federal Agency for Healthcare Research and Quality (AHRQ) is the organization responsible for certifying PSOs, and there are currently approximately 77 federally certified PSOs nationwide.[230] The Act provides federal legal privilege and confidentiality protections to information that is assembled and reported by providers to a PSO or developed by a PSO ("patient safety work product") for the conduct of patient safety activities. Patient safety work product is privileged and not subject to discovery, nor admissible as evidence, in connection with a federal, state, or local civil, criminal, or administrative proceeding, including a proceeding against a medical provider.

6.3 When Are Providers Required or Authorized to Report PHI to Legal Authorities and Others?

Federal and state laws compel disclosure of protected health information in many contexts other than discovery or testimony. Reporting laws have been enacted that require such information to be reported to governmental agencies. The most common examples are vital statistics, infectious diseases, child abuse, and wound reporting laws. Familiarity with these and other reporting laws is important to assure compliance and to avoid reporting to the wrong agency. Reports to the wrong agency may not be legally protected, resulting in potential liability for breach of confidentiality.

HIPAA. The HIPAA Privacy Rule permits covered entities to comply with state laws that require reports or other disclosures.[231]

VITAL STATISTICS. All states require the reporting of births and deaths.[232]

PUBLIC HEALTH. Most states require reports of infectious diseases.[233] A California court observed that in addition to criminal penalties for not reporting, civil liability is possible in a suit by persons who contract diseases that might have been avoided by proper reports.[234] Some states require reports of certain poisonings, cancer cases, and other selected noncontagious diseases.

In 1994, a Missouri appellate court barred enforcement of a local court rule requiring correction facilities to disclose the infectious disease reports of inmates before court appearances.[235]

CHILD ABUSE. All states require reports of suspected cases of child abuse or neglect.[236] The HIPAA Privacy Rule expressly permits child abuse reports.[237]

Some professionals, such as physicians and nurses, are mandatory reporters and thus are required to make reports. Anyone who is not a mandatory reporter may make a report as a permissive reporter. In some states, any report arising out of diagnosis or treatment in an institution must be made through the institutional administration. In some states, a professional is a mandatory reporter only when the child has been examined or treated but is a permissive reporter when the abuse is learned from the abuser or another person.[238] In some states, providers are required to report abuse that they learn from others but only if the abuse occurred in the state.[239]

Most child abuse reporting laws extend some degree of immunity from liability for reports made through proper channels.[240] A mandatory reporter who fails to report child abuse is subject to both criminal penalties[241] and civil liability for future injuries to the child that could have been avoided if a report had been made.[242] In 2003, in a prosecution of an emergency nurse, a Missouri trail court decided that the criminal penalties for not reporting were unconstitutional.[243]

There have been disputes in some states over when some activities, such as sexual activity of younger minors, must be reported as child abuse.[244]

ADULT ABUSE/DOMESTIC VIOLENCE. Some states have enacted adult abuse reporting laws that are similar to the child abuse reporting laws.[245] Unlike child abuse laws, these laws are usually more permissive, with no required reporting.[246] The HIPAA Privacy Rule permits required reports; permissive reports are required in some limited circumstances.[247] These laws are controversial.[248]

WOUNDS. Many states require the reporting of certain wounds.[249] Some states specify that all wounds of certain types must be reported. For example, New York requires the reporting of wounds inflicted by sharp instruments that may result in death and all gunshot wounds.[250] Other states limit the reporting requirement to wounds caused under certain circumstances. For example, Iowa requires the reporting of wounds that apparently resulted from criminal acts.[251]

In 2002, a New York district attorney sought to compel New York City hospitals to produce all records pertaining to male Caucasian emergency room patients between the ages of 30 and 45 who sought treatment for knife wounds on two dates. The highest court of New York ruled that the subpoena could not be enforced. The state law that mandated reporting knife wounds was limited to life-threatening stab wounds. Treatment for other stab wounds was privileged.[252]

DRIVERS. A few states require reports to be submitted to state driver licensing agencies of conditions such as seizures that could lead to loss of license. Most states permit such reports but do not require them.[253]

OTHER REPORTING LAWS. Some states require reports of other information, such as industrial accidents and radiation incidents.[254] National reporting laws apply to hospitals that are involved in manufacturing, testing, or using certain substances and devices. For example, fatalities due to blood transfusions must be reported to the Food and Drug Administration (FDA).[255] A sponsor of an investigational medical device must report to the FDA any unanticipated adverse effects from use of the device.[256] There is a duty to report deaths or serious injuries in connection with devices.[257]

Some states require that major adverse incidents be reported to a state agency.[258] The director of nursing at a nursing home was personally fined in New York for failing to make such a report.[259]

In 1977, the U.S. Supreme Court upheld a state law that required reports to a central state registry of all prescriptions of Schedule II controlled substances.[260]

A federal law requires hospitals to notify emergency transport personnel and other individuals who bring emergency patients to the hospital if the patient is diagnosed as having an infectious disease.[261]

COMMON LAW DUTY TO DISCLOSE. In addition to these statutory requirements, the common law has recognized a duty to disclose medical information in several circumstances. Persons who could have avoided injury if information had been disclosed have won civil suits against providers who failed to disclose such information.

INFECTIOUS DISEASES. When an infectious disease is diagnosed, there is a duty to warn third parties at risk of exposure unless forbidden by statute.[262] However, in most states there is no duty to warn all members of the general public. In a California case, the court observed that liability to the general public might result from failure to make a required report to public health authorities.[263] In at least one state, there is a duty to warn a broader range of individuals. In 1986, the South Carolina Supreme Court ruled that a hospital could be sued by the parents of a girl who had died of meningitis. Her friend had been diagnosed and treated at the hospital for meningitis, and the hospital had not notified persons who had prior contact with its patient during the likely period of contagiousness.[264]

THREATS TO OTHERS. Some courts have ruled that there is a duty to warn identified persons that a patient has made a credible threat to kill them. Other courts have expanded the duty. The first decision to impose this duty was *Tarasoff v. Regents of University of California.*[265] When the Tarasoffs sued for the death of their daughter, the California Supreme Court found the employer of a psychiatrist liable for the psychiatrist's failure to warn the daughter that one of his patients had threatened to kill her. The court ruled that he should have either warned the victim or advised others likely to apprise the victim of the danger. In a 1980 case, the same court clarified the scope of this duty by ruling that only threats to readily identified individuals create a duty to warn, so there is no duty to warn a threatened group.[266]

OTHER DUTIES. Courts have recognized other situations that lead to a duty to disclose. One example is the duty of referral specialists to communicate their findings to the referring physician.[267] A competent patient can waive this duty by directing the referral specialist not to communicate with the referring physician.[268]

6.4 When May Providers Disclose PHI in Response to Inquiries from Legal Authorities?

The HIPAA Privacy Rule authorizes disclosures of PHI without patient authorization for some public health activities,[269] health oversight activities,[270] administrative proceedings,[271] law enforcement purposes,[272] cadaveric organ, eye, or tissue donation purposes,[273] research purposes,[274] to avert a serious threat to health or safety,[275] and various specialized governmental functions. The HIPAA Privacy Rule defines in detail when disclosures without consent can be made for each of these purposes. This section discusses law enforcement disclosures.

PRESENCE IN FACILITY. Providers may confirm the presence in the facility of a named patient or a patient with a physical description (e.g., height, weight, hair and eye color, race, gender, scars, presence or absence of facial hair, scars, and tattoos), except for patients subject to the substance abuse treatment confidentiality rules.[277]

However, generally providers cannot respond to individual law enforcement requests to report when a patient arrives with a particular medical condition. There are at least three exceptions: (1) when the law requires or permits reports about the medical condition (such as certain wounds) to law enforcement; (2) if the law enforcement officer is trying to locate a suspect, victim, or material witness to a crime, in most states providers may disclose type of injury and date and time of treatment or death; or (3) when a law enforcement officer calls to ask for information and discloses that a person who could become a patient is dangerous, providers can take appropriate steps to protect themselves and others from dangerous persons, which in some cases can involve notifying law enforcement officials to assist in protection.

DISCHARGE OF PRISONERS. When persons in law enforcement custody are discharged from the provider back to a jail or prison, generally medical authorities at the jail or prison can be told the information that is necessary for the ongoing care of the prisoner. Guards who are transporting the prisoner generally cannot be told medical information. However, information that is necessary for a safe transport is permitted, for example, a propensity for violence that is not known by the guards.[278]

POLICE REPORTS. Providers are not permitted to provide PHI to law enforcement officers for the purposes of investigating a crime or completing a police report, unless there is written authorization from the patient or court action (search warrant or court order). This includes requests for the extent of injury, diagnoses, treatment plans, personal impressions (e.g., "Did you smell alcohol on his breath?"), and medications. Law enforcement must obtain a search warrant, court order, or patient authorization before accessing PHI. Failure to do so can bar the admissibility of any information obtained.[279] Generally, if a patient has provided false identification to obtain a prescription or other services, information necessary to investigate this crime on the provider's premises can be disclosed to law enforcement.

COLLECTION AND TESTING OF SAMPLES. It is permissible for providers to draw blood and other forensic samples at the request of law enforcement officers to the extent permitted by state law. The most common example of this is the drawing of a blood sample of someone who is suspected of driving while under the influence of alcohol or drugs. Drawing the sample and delivering it to the law enforcement officer for testing by a forensic laboratory is not a disclosure of PHI.

However, providers must not let law enforcement officers influence their decisions whether to draw blood or collect other samples for clinical purposes and testing by the provider. Clinical sample collection at the direction of law enforcement officers can be a constitutional violation, and the results are generally not admissible in court.[280]

When law enforcement officers seek a sample collected for clinical purposes or the results of testing on the sample, they must obtain a court order or search warrant. Providers must not voluntarily release the samples or results. In most states, voluntarily released samples or results generally are not admissible in court.[281]

REMOVAL OF BULLETS AND OTHER FOREIGN OBJECTS. The law concerning removal of bullets or other foreign objects from patients varies somewhat from state to state. There are constitutional limits on compelling such removal (see section 7.4). Assuming the removal is appropriately authorized, there are three approaches to delivering the object to law enforcement. In some circumstances, providers may authorize law enforcement officers to be present during the removal and directly deliver the objects to the witnessing officer without a court order.[282] The circumstances vary from state to state. Wisconsin permits law enforcement officers to be present in the operating room during surgical removal of bags of cocaine if the patient is in law enforcement custody.[283] When law enforcement is not permitted to assume direct custody, the more conservative position is to require a search warrant, court order, or patient consent before releasing objects to law enforcement, but most of the courts that have addressed the question have permitted bullets to be admitted into evidence even when police obtain them without a warrant, order, or consent.[284]

CRIMES ON THE PREMISES. Providers may report crimes that occur on their premises. Usually, disclosure of PHI is not required to make these reports. When PHI is related to the crime, PHI may be disclosed to the extent necessary to provide evidence of the crime. For example, when drugs are stolen, the name and amount of drug may be disclosed, but the diagnosis should generally not be disclosed.

FEDERAL LAW ENFORCEMENT. The HIPAA Privacy Rule permits disclosures for some national security activities and for protective services for the President and others.[285] Disclosures must also be made when necessary for enforcement of the HIPAA Privacy Rules,[286] Medicare, Medicaid, and other governmental payment programs.[287]

6.5 When May Providers Disclose PHI in Response to Inquiries from Others?

Some statutes do not mandate reporting but authorize access to medical records, without the patient's permission, on request of certain individuals or organizations or the general public.

WORKERS' COMPENSATION. Some state statutes grant all parties to a workers' compensation claim access to all relevant medical information after a claim has been made.[288] In some states, courts have ruled that filing a workers' compensation claim is a waiver of confidentiality of relevant medical information.[289] However, in at least one state the physician-patient privilege applies in workers' compensation cases.[290] The HIPAA Privacy Rules permits compliance with these workers' compensation laws.[291]

FEDERAL FREEDOM OF INFORMATION ACT. The federal Freedom of Information Act (FOIA) applies only to federal agencies.[292] A provider does not become a federal agency by receiving federal funds, so the FOIA applies to few hospitals outside of the VA and Defense Department hospital systems. FOIA does not apply to medical files; so disclosure of medical information pursuant to a FOIA request would "constitute a clearly unwarranted invasion of personal privacy." Thus, the FOIA provides only limited protection of confidentiality of medical information in the possession of federal agencies. However, the federal Privacy Act may provide some additional protection to such information.[293]

STATE PUBLIC RECORDS LAWS. Many states have public records laws that apply to state agencies that are covered entities, such as public hospitals. Some state statutes explicitly exempt hospital and medical records from disclosure.[294] In a 1974 case, Colorado's law was interpreted not to permit a publisher to obtain all birth and death reports routinely.[295] In 1983, the Iowa Supreme Court addressed the effort of a leukemia patient to force the disclosure of an unrelated potential bone marrow donor whose name was in the records of a public hospital.[296] The court ruled that names of patients could be withheld from disclosure and that although the potential donor had never sought treatment at the hospital, the potential donor was a patient for purposes of the exemption because the medical procedure of tissue typing had been performed. However, in a 1978 Ohio case, the state law was interpreted to require access to the names and the dates of admission and discharge of all persons admitted to a public hospital.[297] In states that follow the Ohio rule, it is especially important to resist discovery of nonparty records because removal of "identifiers" does not offer much protection when dates in the records may make it possible to identify the patient from the admission list.

OTHER ACCESS LAWS. Some federal and state statutes give governmental agencies access to medical records on request or through administrative subpoena.[298] For example, peer review organizations (PROs) have access to all medical records pertinent to their federal review functions on request. Hospital licensing laws often grant inspectors access without subpoena for audit and inspection purposes.

7 What Legal Issues Flow from the Use of Audio and Video Transmissions and Recordings?

AUDIO RECORDINGS. Federal law and the law of many states permit recording of conversations by any party to the conversation.[299] In most circumstances, the other states require the consent of all parties to the conversation. In some jurisdictions, these laws apply primarily to recording of telephone and other transmitted conversations; in other jurisdictions, they apply to all conversations but generally do not apply where there is no reasonable expectation of privacy.

VISUAL RECORDINGS. Physicians may take and use photographs of patients for the medical record or for professional educational purposes if the patient expressly consents. The Maine Supreme Court ruled that when a patient had expressly objected to being photographed, there could be liability for photographing the patient even if the photograph was solely for the medical record.[300] Liability for photographs taken without express consent is not likely if the patient does not object and uses are appropriately restricted. A New York appellate court ruled that a physician and nurse could not be sued for allowing a newspaper photographer to photograph a patient in the waiting areas of an infectious disease unit because the individual's presence did not indicate the individual was a patient and the individual was never identified as a patient.[301] Public or commercial showing without consent can lead to liability.[302]

Visual recordings have led to a wide variety of situations that courts have addressed. One group of cases deals with the right to make recordings. In 1985, a New York appellate court ruled that representatives of an incompetent patient do not have a right to photograph the patient in the hospital.[303] The petitioners failed to show a sufficient need to justify a court order that they be permitted to film their comatose daughter in an intensive care unit for eight hours for use in a suit. In an unreported New Jersey appellate court case in 2000, a hospital was ordered to permit videotaping in an intensive care unit.[304]

Other suits have dealt with liability for media recordings.[305] In 1998, the California Supreme Court ruled that an accident victim could sue two television production companies for invasion of privacy for taping the victim's medical helicopter flight to the hospital. The court ruled that some of the recording at the scene of the accident may also have constituted an invasion of privacy.[306]

Other suits have involved the use of recordings.[307] In 2002, a Florida trial court permitted the parents of a comatose woman to televise a videotape of her condition since it had been shown in court.[308] In 2002, a woman used the surgeon's videotape of her surgery to support her suit claiming that he had branded her during the surgery.[309]

TJC requires consent before audio or video recording of patients for any purpose other than identification, diagnosis, or treatment.[310] This means that Joint Commission-accredited hospitals must obtain consent for recordings that are for educational purposes.

8 What Legal Issues Flow from the Use of Computers and the Internet?

FEDERAL POLICY. There is an increasing push for use of computerized medical records. In 2004, the President announced an effort to adopt electronic health records by 2014.[311] The Veterans Administration has adopted a computerized medical record.[312] The federal Consolidated Health Informatics Initiative is seeking to establish the framework for sharing health information among federal agencies and is pursuing interoperability standards.[313] An Executive Order in 2004 established a federal Office of Health Information Technology.[314]

The American Relief and Recovery Act of 2009 (ARRA) provides billions of dollars for health information technology investments. Most of the money is available to hospitals and physicians who adopt and meaningfully use qualified electronic health records.

COMPUTERIZED RECORDKEEPING. Computerized records are generally more accessible than paper records for their many functions. Multiple uses can occur concurrently, reducing the need for waiting for others to complete their uses of the paper record. They permit more standardization of datakeeping. They remove some of the problems with legibility of some paper records and assist in reducing some preventable errors. Computer programs can assist physicians in making diagnostic and treatment decisions through clinical decision support. There is an opportunity to build in checking procedures that can call attention to and even bar potentially problematic orders. Computerized records provide an opportunity for more automatic analysis of data.

There are potential disadvantages to computerized systems.[315] Computerized systems are costly.[316] In addition, they can divert professional time from patient care. Data still must be entered by someone. Many approaches require data entry by physicians and other professionals that can divert their time from other functions, reducing the quantity of patient care that can be provided. They create a temptation to require the collection of more data that further diverts resources from

patient care. These are not necessarily arguments against computerization. Rather they need to be kept in mind by those structuring the systems.

Another potential disadvantage is the security risk. Unauthorized users can sometimes gain access. Authorized users can access records for unauthorized purposes. However, this is a strong argument against computerized records. Similar risks exist with paper records. In addition, computerized systems are more effective in tracking uses of records than are paper records. Steps are being taken to provide more security for computerized records.

The HIPAA Privacy and Security Rules apply to access to and use of computerized records. The HIPAA Security Rule requires that computerized records and communications meet basic security standards, effective April 21, 2005.

It is cumbersome to structure computerized records so that authorized persons cannot access records beyond those they need for their job because it is usually not possible to determine in advance which records they will need to access. Thus, training, professional standards, and monitoring of lookups are used to deter and detect inappropriate lookups. There have been few legal cases involving inappropriate lookups.[317]

For several years, some healthcare providers have been developing computerized methods for handling some healthcare information. For a time, one legal barrier was the requirement of authentication of physician entries and orders by a physician signature that could only be performed on a hard copy. Electronic signatures are now generally accepted, so this barrier has largely been removed. In 2000, the federal government adopted a law recognizing electronic signatures for most purposes.[318] However, care must still be exercised in the structuring and use of electronic signatures.[319] Some states have had centralized computer records of some healthcare information. In 1977, the U.S. Supreme Court upheld New York's mandatory reporting of prescriptions, discussing how the information was placed into a centralized state computer system.[320]

Another legal barrier was that some jurisdictions would not accept computerized records as official records. Computerized records are now generally accepted as official records for regulatory and evidentiary purposes if they meet basic standards of reliability.[321]

One barrier to the standardization of documentation has been the difficulty in establishing standard terminology. Progress is being made in addressing this issue. On May 6, 2004, the HHS announced that it had licensed the College of American Pathologists Systematized Nomenclature of Medicine Clinical Terms (SNOMED-CT®) for laboratory result contents, nonlaboratory interventions and procedures, anatomy, diagnosis and problems, and nursing and announced that it was making SNOMED-CT available for use in the United States at no charge to users.[322]

E-MAIL. Many providers use e-mail to communicate with patients and other providers.[323] With appropriate attention to confidentiality and the different nature of interaction, this practice appears to offer advantages. In 1998, a Wisconsin appellate court recognized the validity of e-mail prescriptions.[324] One of the impediments to broader adoption of e-mail communications with patients has been the lack of payment for the time spent in this function.[325] Some payers have experimented with payments.[326]

E-mail communications should be treated with the same degree of care and formality as other written communications. They can be discovered and used in criminal investigations and civil lawsuits.[327] Federal courts have generally determined that they are not subject to the same degree of protection as telephone calls, so it may not be a violation of federal wiretap laws to intercept e-mail at several stages in their transmission.[328] Some employers have increased the monitoring of e-mail and other computer use.[329]

E-mail is also sometimes used for threats and harassment.[330]

Care must be taken when sending e-mail in a healthcare environment. There have been a few incidents where medical information was accidentally distributed to the wrong recipients.[331] The HIPAA security rules apply to e-mail and will require encryption and other steps to improve the security of e-mail.

INTERNET. Computerized records have been stolen through the Internet.[332] It is important for those responsible for computers to monitor and implement security precautions.[333]

Computerized records have been accidentally posted on the Internet.[334] It is important to train staff on how to minimize these accidents.

There have been challenges to postings on the Internet. In 1999, a jury awarded $107 million verdict against an antiabortion group who had produced wanted posters of abortion providers and had supplied then to a website.

The trial court enjoined production of the posters and the supplying of them to the website. A federal appellate court upheld the injunction and the verdict against the group but required that the lower court review the amount of the judgment. The appellate court found that there was a sufficient threat of force on the posters to overcome the First Amendment protection for the posters. In 2004, the lower court affirmed the amount of the judgment.[335] In 2001, another antiabortion group created a website that includes photographs and medical records of women who had obtained abortions. A Missouri state lower court enjoined removal of the photographs and records.[336]

In 2002, a Massachusetts court required a patient to remove misleading photos and defamatory statements from a website about a physician.[337] In 2003, a Pennsylvania judge ordered attorneys to close a website for recruiting patients for a class action lawsuit, but it was reopened later after a settlement with the hospital that involved deleting the hospital's name from the website name.[338]

SOCIAL MEDIA. Social media has invaded health care from at least three fronts: innovative startups, patient communities, and medical centers. Patient communities are flourishing in an environment rich with social networks, both through mainline social communities and condition-specific communities. Meanwhile, hospitals and academic medical centers are diving into the social media mix with YouTube channels, Facebook pages, and Twitter accounts.

At the same time, healthcare organizations find challenges in adopting social media. Hospitals and medical practices are risk adverse and generally cautious about new technology trends without clear value. There are questions about whether social media use by hospital employees is a waste of time, or even worse, presents risks of violating HIPAA or leaking proprietary information. Hospital IT departments are concerned about security risks. Individual privacy concerns, particularly the vulnerability of social media accounts, are also cited as a reason to avoid social media in a healthcare setting.

Whether interacting with patients and their healthcare information in person or digitally via the Internet or other social media outlets, providers should always respect patient confidentiality and take care to maintain the security of healthcare information.

Chapter Summary

Medical research increases the body of available clinical data about patients (e.g., genetics data, hormone levels, neurological impairment) while the Internet grows the risk of disclosure of such data exponentially. Access to "private" health information is subject to laws and regulations, which inevitably trail advances in medical research and computing technology. In the United States, efforts to target marketing to individuals utilizing their private health information are pushing the boundaries of applicable law and are past the boundaries applied in the European Union. Debates on the protections that should be applied to private health information are informed by the breadth and scope of law and regulations reviewed in this chapter. The law related to the intersection of private health information with computers, e-mail, social media, and the Internet is still developing. It can be anticipated that new legal issues will continue to flow from this changing area.

Key Terms and Definitions

Healthcare Information – Broadly defined, is aggregate and individually specific patient data including personal information (such as name, date of birth, sex, marital status, occupation, next of kin, etc.), financial information (such as employer, health insurance identification number, and other information to assist in billing), and medical history (such as physical examinations, diagnoses, treatment recommendations and treatment administered, progress reports, physician orders, clinical laboratory results, radiology reports, nursing notes, discharge summaries, etc.).

Medical Records – Created when a person receives treatment from a health professional and includes personal, financial, and medical data.

ARRA – The acronym for the American Recovery and Reinvestment Act of 2009, the economic stimulus package passed by the U.S. Congress and signed into law by President Obama in February 2009. ARRA provided billions of dollars of incentives, in the form of reimbursement, to assist and encourage doctors and hospitals to transition away from the maintenance of paper medical records and adopt electronic health records.

NGO – The abbreviation for nongovernmental organization. NGOs operate independently from federal and state governments. NGOs may receive governmental financial support but maintain their independence by excluding government from NGO membership and management. The Joint Commission is an example of an NGO.

The Joint Commission (TJC) – An independent, not-for-profit organization that accredits and certifies healthcare organizations and programs in the United States. The Joint Commission accreditation and certification is a recognized symbol of quality that reflects an organization's commitment to certain performance standards. To be accredited, hospitals must meet The Joint Commission medical records standards. To earn and maintain The Joint Commission accreditation submission to periodic on-site survey by a Joint Commission survey team is required.

CMS – The acronym for the Centers for Medicare & Medicaid Services, the branch of the U.S. Department of Health and Human Services that administers Medicare and Medicaid.

Medicare – The U.S. government's national health insurance program for people 65 years or older and under age 65 with certain disabilities.

Medicaid – A jointly funded, federal-state health insurance program for low-income and needy people.

HHS – The acronym for the Department of Health and Human Services, the U.S. government's principal agency for protecting the health of all Americans and providing essential human services.

HIPAA – The acronym for the Health Insurance Portability and Accountability Act of 1996, enacted by the U.S. Congress and signed by President Clinton. Title II of HIPAA directed HHS to draft rules establishing national security and privacy health data standards.

Covered Entities – Healthcare clearinghouses, employer-sponsored health plans, health insurers, and medical service providers to which the HIPAA privacy and security rules regulating protected health information apply.

Business Associates - Independent contractors who engage in business with or otherwise assist covered entities and have access to protected health information.

Protected Health Information - Any information held by a covered entity or its business associates that concerns health status, the provision of health care, or payment for health care and can be linked to an individual.

HHS Office for Civil Rights - Enforces the HIPAA Privacy and Security Rules.

Office of the National Coordinator for Health Information Technology - Organizationally located within HHS and is the principal Federal entity charged with coordinating nationwide efforts to implement and use advanced health information technology and electronic exchange of health information.

HIPAA Privacy Rule - Establishes national standards to protect medical records and other personal health information. It requires covered entities and their business associates to protect the privacy of personal health information and sets limits and conditions on the uses and disclosures that may be made of such information without patient authorization. It also gives patients rights over their health information, including rights to examine and obtain a copy of their health records, and to request corrections.

HIPAA Security Rule - Establishes national standards to protect individuals' electronic personal health information that is created, received, used, or maintained by a covered entity. It requires appropriate administrative, physical and technical safeguards to ensure the confidentiality, integrity, and security of electronic protected health information.

Instructor-Led Questions

1. What are some of the underlying issues that must be balanced in developing laws and policies concerning healthcare information?

2. Who owns the medical record?

3. What information must be collected in a medical record?

4. How should a provider determine how long to keep medical records?

5. What are the basic HIPAA requirements concerning privacy of protected healthcare information?

6. Which state laws are still in effect? What other federal privacy laws remain in effect?

7. When may patients and their representatives authorize disclosure?

8. When may the law compel disclosure?

9. When are reports to legal authorities required?

10. When may providers release information in response to requests from others?

11. Has HIPAA struck the proper balance between privacy and uses of healthcare information?

12. What restrictions are there on audio and video recordings in healthcare settings?

13. What are some of the legal issues related to the use of computers and the Internet in health care?

14. What are some of the advantages and disadvantages of computerized medical records?

Endnotes

1 Inside trader avoids prison, N.Y. Times, Jan. 16, 1999, A16 [convicted lawyer given no prison sentence because his cerebral palsy made him vulnerable to prison hardships].

2 See Massachusetts board probes shared Rx information, Am. Med. News, May 25, 1998, 13 [sharing prescription drug information with marketing company]; *Legal Economic Evaluations v. Metropolitan Life Ins. Co.*, 39 F.3d 951 (9th Cir. 1994), cert. denied, 514 U.S. 1044 (1995) [summary judgment for defendants in suit by consultants who provided services to tort claimants on costs of structured settlements, not antitrust violation for life insurance companies to refuse to provide information other than for defense].

3 E.g., *Pyramid Life Ins. Co. v. Masonic Hosp. Ass'n*, 191 F. Supp. 51 (W.D. Okla. 1961); see also *Archive America, Inc. v. Variety Children's Hosp.*, 873 So. 2d 359 (Fla. 3d Dist. 2004) [warehouseman's lien transferred from stored hospital records to bond].

4 But see *University of Tex. Med. Branch v. York*, 871 S.W.2d 175 (Tex. 1994) [medical record not tangible personal property; information intangible, fact of recordation does not render information tangible].

5 E.g., *Cannell v. Medical & Surg. Clinic*, 21 Ill. App. 3d 383, 315 N.E.2d 278 (3d Dist. 1974).

6   *Cornelio v. Stamford Hosp.*, 246 Conn. 45, 717 A.2d 140 (1998); *Lucarello v. North Shore Univ. Hosp.*, 184 A.D.2d 623, 584 N.Y.S.2d 906 (2d Dept. 1992).

7   E.g., *McGarry v. J. A. Mercier Co.*, 272 Mich. 501, 262 N.W. 296 (1935); Gerson v. New York Women's Medical, 249 A.D.2d 265, 671 N.Y.S.2d 104 (2d Dept. 1998) [provider owns mammogram films].

8   E.g., *Caldwell v. Shalala*, 114 F.3d 216 (D.C. Cir.), cert. denied, 522 U.S. 916 (1997) [physician with conditionally reinstated privileges at Army hospital entitled to access medical records].

9   E.g., *Simmons v. Southwest Florida Reg. Med. Ctr.*, No. 98-2046 CA RWP (Fla. Cir. Ct. Lee County Apr. 24, 1998), as discussed in 26 Health L. Dig. (July 1998), 57 [office-generated patient medical records developed by physicians while employed by hospital belong to physicians not hospital that terminated them]; State ex rel. O'Donnell v. Clifford, 948 S.W.2d 451 (Mo. Ct. App. 1997) [per written employment agreement, terminated physician entitled to copy medical records of patients he had treated only on request by patient].

10   42 C.F.R. § 482.24(c).

11   Joint Commission, 2011 Comprehensive Accreditation Manual for Hospitals, Elements of Performance for RC.01.01.01 [hereinafter 2011 JC CAMH].

12   E.g., J. Olson, Pediatrician loses license for failure to keep up records, Omaha World Herald, Mar. 18, 2002, 5B.

13   *Nassau County Med. Ctr. v. Zinman* (N.Y. Dist. Ct. Aug. 1998), as discussed in N.Y. L.J, Aug. 3, 1998, 25.

14   E.g., *Valendon Martinez v. Hospital Presbiteriano de la Communidad, Inc.*, 806 F.2d 1128 (1st Cir. 1986).

15   *Lama v. Borras*, 16 F.3d 473 (1st Cir. 1994).

16   *Repp v. Anadarko Municipal Hosp.*, 43 F.3d 519 (10th Cir. 1994).

17   E.g., M. Greenberg, Writer's cramp has reached epidemic levels, Am. Med. News, Aug. 3, 1998, 18 [documentation requirements for referrals]; Budget-killer progress notes tamed, Am. Med. News, Feb.1, 1999, 18.

18   2011 JC CAMH, RC.01.01.01.

19   *Hiatt v. Groce*, 215 Kan. 14, 523 P.2d 320 (1974).

20   *Collins v. Westlake Commun. Hosp.*, 57 Ill. 2d 388, 312 N.E.2d 614 (1974).

21   *Sunnen v. Administrative Review Bd.*, 244 A.D.2d 790, 666 N.Y.S.2d 239 (3d Dept. 1997).

22   *Illiano v. Seaview Orthopedics*, 299 N.J. Super. 99, 690 A.2d 662 (App. Div. 1997).

23   *Engle v. Clarke*, 346 S.W.2d 13 (Ky. 1961); contra *Thome v. Palmer*, 141 Ill. App. 3d 92, 489 N.E.2d 1163 (3d Dist. 1986); *Hurlock v. Park Lane Med. Ctr.*, 709 S.W.2d 872 (Mo. Ct. App. 1985).

24   42 C.F.R. § 482.24(c)(2)(viii).

25   2011 JC CAMH at Elements of Performance RC.01.03.01.

26   E.g., *Board of Trustees v. Pratt*, 72 Wyo. 120, 262 P.2d 682 (1953). Some hospitals use financial incentives, E.g., Incentives spur physicians to complete record-keeping, Mod. Healthcare, Dec. 6, 1985, 64; L. Perry, Emphasis on coordination hastens submission of bills, Mod. Healthcare, July 14, 1989, 39.

27   *Birthisel v. Tri-Cities Health Services Corp.*, 188 W.Va. 371, 424 S.E.2d 606 (1992).

28   42 C.F.R. § 482.24(c)(1); 2011 JC CAMH at Elements of Performance RC.01.04.01 and MS.05.01.03.

29   *Manso-Pizarro v. Secretary of Health & Human Servs.*, 76 F.3d 15 (1st Cir. 1996).

30   *Eldridge v. Metropolitan Life Ins. Co.*, 123 F.3d 456 (7th Cir. 1997).

31   Misread prescription brings $450K award, National L. J., Nov. 8, 1999, A4.

32   R.A. Friedman, Do spelling and penmanship count? In medicine, you bet, N.Y. Times, Mar. 11, 2003, D5.

33   § 456.42, Fla. Stat.; D. Adams, Florida tells doctors: Print clearly or else, Am. Med. News, Aug. 4, 2003, 1; see also Rev. Code Wash. § 69.41.120 [requiring legible prescriptions].

34   Doctor blames poor penmanship for losing license, AP, Feb. 8, 2003.

35   E.g., *Humphreys v. Drug Enforcement Admin.*, 105 F.3d 112 (3d Cir. 1996) [DEA should not have revoked physician's registration to distribute controlled substances for prescribed drugs for famous patient in another's name to protect patient's privacy].

36   *Kaplan v. Central Med. Group*, 71 A.D.2d 912, 419 N.Y.S.2d 750 (2d Dept. 1979).

37   *Murkin v. Medical Mut. Liability Ins. Society*, 82 Md. App. 540, 572 A.2d 1126 (1990).

38   E.g., *Vest v. United States*, 116 F.3d 1179 (7th Cir. 1997), cert. denied, 522 U.S. 1119 (1998) [affirming physician mail fraud conviction for falsifying medical records, ordering unnecessary procedures]; Dentist pays for altering records, AP, Jan. 7, 2003 [Idaho MD sentenced to 10 months home confinement for altering records to obstruct Medicaid fraud investigation]; Waterbury Hospital fined in audit scandal, AP, Mar. 4, 2003 [Conn. hosp. staff added treatment plans and signatures to records selected by federal auditors].

39   E.g., *Tang v. De Buono*, 235 A.D.2d 745, 652 N.Y.S.2d 408 (3d Dept. 1997) [upholding revoking medical license for falsifying CT scan report for insurance fraud]; *Jimenez v. Department of Professional Reg.*, 556 So. 2d 1219 (Fla. 4th DCA 1990) [one-year suspension of physician's license, $5,000 fine, and two years' probation after suspension for adding false information to records after death of patient]; Doctor fined in teen's death to keep license, Palm Beach (Fla.) Post, Aug. 6, 1995, 23A [violated state law by ordering partner to falsify medical records; fine, probation, community service].

40   *Stevenson v. Comm.*, 27 Va. Ct. App. 453, 499 S.E.2d 580 (1998), aff'd without op. en banc by equally divided court, 28 Va. Ct. App. 562, 507 S.E.2d 625 (1998).

41 E.g., In re Morris, 482 A.2d 369 (D.C. 1984); see also *Caraballo v. Secretary of HHS*, 670 F. Supp. 1106 (D. P.R. 1987) [judicially altered birth certificate not conclusive evidence of age].

42 42 C.F.R. § 482.24(b)(1).

43 42 U.S.C. § 1395x(v)(1)(I).

44 *Bondu v. Gurvich*, 473 So. 2d 1307 (Fla. 3d DCA 1984); *DeLaughter v. Lawrence County Hosp.*, 601 So. 2d 818 (Miss. 1992) [missing records create rebuttable adverse presumption]; *Phillips v. Covenant Clinic*, 625 N.W.2d 714 (Iowa 2001) [can create inference but not in this case]; Annotation, Medical malpractice: presumption or inference from failure of hospital or doctor to produce relevant medical records, 69 A.L.R. 4TH 906.

45 E.g., *Ortega v. Trevino*, 938 S.W.2d 219 (Tex. Ct. App. 1997); *Holmes v. Amerex Rent-A-Car*, 710 A.2d 846 (D.C. App. 1998).

46 E.g., *Miller v. Gupta*, 174 Ill. 2d 120, 672 N.E.2d 1229 (1996) [lost X-ray; duty to preserve evidence can only arise from agreement, contract, statute, or special circumstance].

47 E.g., *Fletcher v. Dorchester Mut. Ins. Co.*, 437 Mass. 544, 773 N.E.2d 420 (2002); *Temple Comm. Hosp. v. Superior Court*, 20 Cal. 4th 464, 976 P.2d 223, 84 Cal. Rptr. 2d 852 (1999); *Goff v. Harold Ives Trucking Co. Inc.*, 27 S.W.3d 387 (Ark. 2000); *Meyn v. State*, 594 N.W.2d 31 (Iowa 1999); see also *Keene v. Brigham & Women's Hosp.*, 439 Mass. 223, 786 N.E.2d 824 (2003) [trial court cannot bypass rejection of separate spoliation action by imposing a default against hospital].

48 *Elmer v. Tenneco Resins, Inc.*, 698 F. Supp. 535 (D. Del. 1988).

49 E.g., TENN. CODE ANN. § 68-11-305(c).

50 *Palmer v. New York State Dep't of Mental Hygiene*, 44 N.Y.2d 958, 408 N.Y.S.2d 322, 380 N.E.2d 154 (1978).

51 *Wolfe v. Beal*, 477 Pa. 447, 384 A.2d 1187 (1978).

52 PUB. L. 104-191, §§ 264(b), (c)(1) (1996).

53 65 FED. REG. 82,461 (Dec. 28, 2000).

54 67 FED. REG. 53,181 (Aug. 14, 2002), codified as 45 C.F.R. Parts 160, 164, Subparts A, E.

55 *South Carolina Med. Ass'n v. Thompson*, 327 F.3d 346 (4th Cir. 2003), cert. denied, 540 U.S. 981 (2003) [initial rule]; *Association of Am. Physicians & Surgeons v. U.S. D.H.H.S.*, 224 F. Supp .2d 1115 (S.D. Tex. 2002) [initial rule]; *Citizens for Health v. Thompson*, 2004 U.S. Dist. LEXIS 5745 (E.D. Pa.) [amended rule] app'd, 2005 U.S. App. LEXIS 23516 (3d Cir).

56 45 C.F.R. §§ 164.500, et seq.

57 45 C.F.R. §§ 160.102, 160.103.

58 45 C.F.R. §§ 164.500, et seq.

59 Id.

60 45 C.F.R. §§ 164.500(a), 160.103 ["health information"], 164.501 ["individually identifiable health information," "protected health information"].

61 45 C.F.R. § 164.520.

62 45 C.F.R. § 164.530.

63 45 C.F.R. § 164.506.

64 45 C.F.R. § 164.512.

65 45 C.F.R. § 164.510(a).

66 45 C.F.R. § 164.502(b).

67 45 C.F.R. § 164.522(b).

68 45 C.F.R. § 164.524.

69 45 C.F.R. § 164.526.

70 45 C.F.R. § 164.528.

71 45 C.F.R. § 164.522.

72 45 C.F.R. §§ 164.502(e), 164.504(e).

73 45 C.F.R. § 164.530.

74 45 C.F.R. § 164.514(e), (f).

75 http://www.hhs.gov/ocr/privacy/hipaa/enforcement/highlights/index.html

76 Privacy complaints filed with HHS show confusion over rule's scope, requirements, HEALTH LAW RPTR. [BNA], Feb. 26, 2004, 282 [4266 complaints−41% closed]; No prosecutions yet under privacy rule, intent to sell, profit key factors in decision, HEALTH LAW RPTR. [BNA], Mar. 11, 2004, 356.

77 P. Shukovsky, Hospitalized man catches identity thief, ex-lab tech pleads guilty to using private health files, credit cards, SEATTLE POST-INTELLIGENCER, Aug. 20, 2004, B1; First sentence for violating privacy act, N.Y. TIMES, Nov. 7, 2004, 22 [16-month sentence].

78 R. Pear, Ruling limits prosecutions of people who violate law on privacy of medical records, N.Y. TIMES, June 7, 2005, 16. The DOJ memo appears at http://www.justice.gov/olc/hipaa_final.htm [accessed Mar. 4, 2012].

79 E.g, *Univ. of Colo. Hosp. Auth. v. Denver Publ. Co.*, 340 F. Supp. 2d 1142 (D. Colo. 2004).

80 45 C.F.R. §§ 160.201-160.205.

81 E.g., Former Houston hospital worker arrested for stealing, selling patient records, AP, Aug. 28, 2003 [patient care assistant sold records to investigator].

82 *Sassali v. Rockford Mem. Hosp.*, 296 Ill. App. 3d 80, 693 N.E.2d 1287 (2d Dist 1998).

83 *Hahnemann Univ. Hosp. v. Edgar*, 74 F.3d 456 (3d Cir. 1996).

84 E.g., FLA. STAT. § 381.609(2)(f) [AIDS], § 455.2416 [permitting disclosure of AIDS to sexual partner, needle-sharing partner]; *Woods v. White*, 689 F. Supp. 874 (W.D. Wis. 1988), aff'd without op., 899 F.2d 17 (7th Cir. 1990) [prisoner could sue staff for disclosing AIDS test to other prisoners]; Annotation, Validity, construction, and effect of state statutes or regulations expressly governing disclosure of fact that person has tested positive for acquired immunodeficiency syndrome (AIDS), 12 A.L.R. 5th 149.

85 F.W. Hafferty, A new MD "nightmare": HIV status disclosure can mean lawsuits for breach of confidentiality, Am. Med. News, Nov. 4, 1988, 27.

86 *Doe v. Roe*, 155 Misc. 2d 392, 588 N.Y.S.2d 236 (Sup. Ct. 1992), modified & aff'd, 190 A.D.2d 463, 599 N.Y.S.2d 350 (4th Dept. 1993).

87 *Nolley v. County of Erie*, 776 F. Supp. 715 (W.D. N.Y. 1991).

88 *Suesbury v. Caceres*, 840 A.2d 1285 (D.C. App. 2004).

89 In re Milton S. Hershey Med. Ctr., 535 Pa. 9, 634 A.2d 159 (1993).

90 *Weston v. Carolina Medicorp, Inc.*, 102 N.C. App. 370, 402 S.E.2d 653 (1991).

91 E.g., D. Shelton, Naming names, Am. Med. News, Apr. 6, 1998, 11 [Illinois becomes 32nd state to require reporting names of HIV-positive persons]; L. Richardson, New York state sets regulations on H.I.V. reporting and partner notification, N.Y. Times, Mar. 13, 1999, A13; H.I.V. secrecy is proving deadly, N.Y. Times, Nov. 25, 2003, F6 [failure to disclose to partners is factor in spreading HIV].

92 E.g., *Boyd v. Wynn*, 286 Ky. 173, 150 S.W.2d 648 (1941).

93 Annotation, Physician's tort liability for unauthorized disclosure of confidential information about patient, 48 A.L.R. 4th 668.

94 *Doe v. Roe*, 93 Misc. 2d 201, 400 N.Y.S.2d 668 (Sup. Ct. 1977).

95 *Humphers v. First Interstate Bank*, 298 Or. 706, 696 P.2d 527 (1985).

96 E.g., *Simonsen v. Swenson*, 104 Neb. 224, 177 N.W. 831 (1920) [physician]; *Knecht v. Vandalia Med. Ctr., Inc.*, 14 Ohio App. 3d 129, 470 N.E.2d 230 (1984) [receptionist].

97 E.g., *Crippen v. Charter Southland Hosp.*, 534 So. 2d 286 (Ala 1988) [disclosure to employer's psychiatrist]; *Tower v. Hirshhorn*, 397 Mass. 581, 492 N.E.2d 728 (1986) [disclosure to insurer's physician].

98 *Horne v. Patton*, 291 Ala. 701, 287 So. 2d 824 (1973).

99 E.g., *Alberts v. Devine*, 395 Mass. 59, 479 N.E.2d 113, cert. denied, 474 U.S. 1013 (1985).

100 *Clark v. Geraci*, 29 Misc. 2d 791, 208 N.Y.S.2d 564 (Sup. Ct. 1960).

101 E.g., *Thomas v. Hillson*, 184 Ga. App. 302, 361 S.E.2d 278 (1987); see Annotation, Libel and slander: privilege of statements by physician, surgeon, or nurse concerning patient, 73 A.L.R. 2D 325.

102 E.g., *Beatty v. Baston*, 130 Ohio L. Abs. 481 (Ct. App. 1932).

103 *United States v. Willis*, 778 F. Supp. 205 (S.D. N.Y. 1991), 737 F. Supp. 269 (1990); Psychiatrist is sentenced, N.Y. Times, Jan. 8, 1992, C12.

104 E.g., *Brand v. Seider*, 697 A.2d 846 (Me. 1997) [claim against psychiatrist alleging breach of confidentiality subject to state malpractice act; contra *Champion v. Cox*, 689 So. 2d 365 (Fla. 1st DCA 1997) [defamation action based upon medical disclosure to patient's employer not subject to state malpractice act].

105 *Allred v. State*, 554 P.2d 411 (Alaska 1976).

106 Fed. R. Evid. 501; *United States v. Bercier*, 848 F.2d 917 (8th Cir. 1988) [criminal]; *United States v. Moore*, 970 F.2d 48 (5th Cir. 1992) [IRS summons]; see Annotation, Situations in which federal courts are governed by state law of privilege under Rule 501 of Federal Rules of Evidence, 48 A.L.R. Fed. 259.

107 E.g., *Roosevelt Hotel Ltd. Partnership v. Sweeney*, 394 N.W.2d 353 (Iowa 1986).

108 Pa. Stat. Ann. title. 42, § 5929; In re June 1979 Allegheny County Investigating Grand Jury, 490 Pa. 143, 415 A.2d 73 (1980).

109 Kan. Stat. Ann. § 60-427.

110 Mich. Comp. Laws § 600.2157.

111 N.Y. Civil Practice L. & R. § 4504.

112 E.g., In re *New York City Council v. Goldwater*, 284 N.Y. 296, 31 N.E.2d 31 (1940).

113 E.g., *Edelstein v. Department of Public Health*, 240 Conn. 658, 692 A.2d 803 (1997) [physician-patient privilege not applicable to subpoena by state public health department investigating billing practices].

114 *Wiles v. Wiles*, 264 Ga. 594, 448 S.E.2d 681 (1994).

115 *Jaffee v. Redmund*, 518 U.S. 1 (1996); *Newton v. Kemna*, 354 F.3d 776 (8th Cir. 2004) [denied access to challenge competency of witness]; *Oleszko v. State Comp. Ins. Fund*, 243 F.3d 1154 (9th Cir. 2001) [Employee Assistance Program information protected]; *Henry v. Kernan*, 197 F.3d 1021 (9th Cir. 1999) [must have reasonable belief doctor is psychotherapist for privilege to apply]; *United States v. Schwensow*, 151 F.3d 650 (7th Cir. 1998) [communications with the Alcoholics Anonymous telephone hotline volunteers not protected, since not psychotherapists].

116 E.g., *United States v. Chase*, 340 F.3d 978 (9th Cir. 2003) (en banc), cert. denied, 540 U.S. 1220 (2004); *United States v. Hayes*, 227 F.3d 578 (6th Cir 2000); *United States v. Glass*, 133 F.3d 1356 (10th Cir. 1998) [refuse to apply dangerous patient exception to facts of case]: but see also In re Grand Jury Proceedings (Violette), 183 F.3d 71 (1st Cir. 1999) [crime-fraud exception recognized].

117 *Schoffstall v. Henderson*, 223 F.3d 818 (8th Cir. 2000); contra, *Vanderbilt v. Town of Chilmark*, 174 F.R.D. 225, 225-30 (D. Mass. 1997) (declining to find waiver where plaintiff sought emotional distress damages).

118 See Medical records increasingly open, Wis. St. J., May 26, 1997, 3B.

119 E.g., *Inabnit v. Berkson*, 199 Cal. App. 3d 1230, 245 Cal. Rptr. 525 (5th Dist. 1988) [patient's failure to challenge subpoena waived privilege].

120 E.g., *Cartwright v. Maccabees Mut. Life Ins. Co.*, 65 Mich. App. 670, 238 N.W.2d 368 (1975), rev'd on other grounds, 398 Mich. 238, 247 N.W.2d 298 (1976) [when misrepresentations in insurance application, life insurer entitled to verdict when widow invoked privilege].

121 E.g., *Willis v. Order of R.R. Telegraphers*, 139 Neb. 46, 296 N.W. 443 (1941).

122 *United States v. Bishop*, 1998 U.S. App. LEXIS 15147 (6th Cir.) [conviction for murdering fellow VA patient upheld; disclosure to police permitted therapists to testify].

123 E.g., *Maynard v. City of San Jose*, 37 F.3d 1396 (9th Cir. 1994); *Premack v. J.C.J. Ogar, Inc.*, 148 F.R.D. 140 (E.D. Pa. 1993).

124 E.g., *Sykes v. St. Andrews School*, 619 So. 2d 467 (Fla. 4th DCA 1993).

125 E.g., State ex rel. *Kitzmiller v. Henning*, 190 W.Va. 142, 437 S.W.2d 452 (1993); *McClelland v. Ozenberger*, 841 S.W.2d 227 (Mo. Ct. App. 1992); *Loudon v. Mhyre*, 110 Wash. 2d 675, 756 P.2d 138 (1988); *Nelson v. Lewis*, 130 N.H. 106, 534 A.2d 720 (1987).

126 E.g., *Huzjak v. United States*, 118 F.R.D. 61 (N.D. Ohio 1987) [treating physician may voluntarily engage in ex parte contacts, but cannot be compelled to do so]; *Trans-World Invs. v. Drobny*, 554 P.2d 1148 (Alaska 1976); *Gobuty v. Kavanagh*, 795 F. Supp. 281 (D. Minn. 1992) [state law permitted defending physician to informally communicate with plaintiff's treating physician with 15 days' notice].

127 E.g., *Requena v. Franciscan Sisters Health Care Corp.*, 212 Ill. App. 3d 328, 570 N.E.2d 1214 (3d Dist. 1991).

128 *Law v. Zuckerman*, 307 F. Supp. 2d 705 (D. Md. 2004) [HIPAA precludes ex parte contacts with treating MD].

129 42 C.F.R. pt. 2, implementing 42 U.S.C § 290dd-2.

130 *Center for Legal Advocacy v. Earnest*, 320 F.3d 1107 (10th Cir. 2003); 59 FED. REG. 42,561 (Aug. 18, 1994).

131 E.g., United States ex rel. *Chandler v. Cook County*, 277 F.3d 969 (7th Cir. 2002) [mandamus striking down discovery order contrary to regulations].

132 E.g., *United States v. Hopper*, 440 F. Supp. 1208 (N.D. Ill. 1977) [probation revocation]; In re Baby X, 97 Mich. App. 111, 293 N.W.2d 736 (1980) [child neglect]; see also *United States v. Corona*, 849 F.2d 562 (11th Cir. 1988), cert. denied, 489 U.S. 1084 (1989) [trial court did not err in permitting use of records of defendant when court could have found criteria for disclosure met].

133 *United States v. Providence Hosp.*, 507 F. Supp. 519 (E.D. Mich. 1981).

134 E.g., In re August, 1993 Regular Grand Jury, 854 F. Supp. 1380 (S.D. Ind. 1994) [grand jury investigation of possible criminal conduct by psychotherapist]; *State Bd. of Medical Examiners v. Fenwick Hall, Inc.*, 308 S.C. 477, 419 S.E.2d 222 (1992) [disclosure to licensing board]; *O'Boyle v. Jensen*, 150 F.R.D. 519 (M.D. Pa. 1993) [civil rights suit for death in police custody].

135 E.g., *United States v. Cresta*, 825 F.2d 538 (1st Cir. 1987), cert. denied, 486 U.S. 1042 (1988) [credibility]; *United States v. Smith*, 789 F.2d 196 (3d Cir. 1986) [credibility]; D. Canedy, Judge upholds privacy for Jeb Bush's daughter, N.Y. TIMES, Oct. 1, 2002, A22 [drug possession investigation].

136 E.g., *Ellison v. Cocke County, Tenn.*, 63 F.3d 467 (6th Cir. 1995); *Chapa v. Adams*, 168 F.3d 1036 (7th Cir. 1999); *Doe v. Broderick*, 225 F.3d 2000 (4th Cir. 2000).

137 20 U.S.C. § 1232g(d).

138 See S. Tavernise, In college and in despair, with parents in the dark, N.Y. TIMES, Oct. 26, 2003, 1.

139 45 C.F.R. 164.501 ["protected health information"].

140 15 U.S.C. 1681b(g); D. Paletta, Medical data rules: exceptions proposed, AM. BANKER, Apr. 7, 2004, 4; 69 FED. REG. 23,380 (Apr. 28, 2004) [proposed rules].

141 5 U.S.C. § 552a.

142 45 C.F.R. §§ 160.103 ["health care"], 164.501 ["treatment"].

143 E.g., *Wilkinson v. Methodist*, Richard Young Hosp., 259 Neb. 745, 612 N.W.2d 213 (2000) [hospital staff may access, use computer information for billing purposes].

144 45 C.F.R. § 164.501 ["payment"].

145 45 C.F.R. § 164.501 ["health care operations"].

146 *Hyman v. Jewish Chronic Disease Hosp.*, 15 N.Y.2d 317, 258 N.Y.S.2d 397, 399, 206 N.E.2d 338 (1965).

147 *Klinge v. Lutheran Med. Ctr.*, 518 S.W.2d 157 (Mo. Ct. App. 1974).

148 In re General Accident Assurance Co. of Canada & Sunnybrook Hosp., 23 O.R.(2d) 513 (Ont. High Ct. of Justice 1979); accord *Rea v. Pardo*, 132 A.D.2d 442, 522 N.Y.S.2d 393 (4th Dept. 1987) [patient request to send record to attorney justified physician sending copy to his insurer]; *Archambault v. Roller*, 254 Va. 210, 491 S.E.2d 729 (1997) [nonparty physician being deposed in malpractice action may disclose patient information to attorney].

149 *Biddle v. Warren Gen. Hosp.*, 86 Ohio St. 3d 395, 715 N.E.2d 518 (1999).

150 E.g., *Lancaster v. Loyola Univ. Med. Ctr.*, 1992 U.S. Dist. LEXIS 15207 (N.D. Ill.) [hospital employees]; *Morgan v. Cook County*, 252 Ill. App. 3d 947, 625 N.E.2d 136 (1st Dist. 1993) [treating physician, when suit seeks to make hospital vicariously liable]; *Alachua Gen. Hosp. v. Stewart*, 649 So. 2d 357 (Fla. 1st DCA 1995) [physician, when suit seeks to make hospital vicariously liable]; but see *Ritter v. Rush-Presbyterian-St. Luke's Med. Ctr.*, 177 Ill. App. 3d 313, 532 N.E.2d 327 (1st Dist. 1988) [hospital not even permitted to interview its codefendant employee treating physicians].

151 45 C.F.R. § 46.101(b)(5); 46 FED. REG. 8,392 (1981); see also 56 FED. REG. 67,078 (1991) [HCFA allowed release of patient identifiable information from Uniform Clinical Data Set for research purposes].

152 See, E.g., T. Meyer, Chest radiation linked to breast cancer, WIS. ST. J., Feb. 13, 1998, 6A [discovery from review of medical records of 3,436 patients]; D. McKenzie, Harvesting data: A little less privacy leads to better care, AM. MED. NEWS, Jan. 26, 1998, 14; Scientists use medical-record data bases to detect adverse side effects of drugs, WALL ST. J., Mar. 24, 1988, 33; L. Gordis & E. Gold, Privacy, confidentiality, and the use of medical records in research, 207 SCIENCE 153 (1980).

153 45 C.F.R. § 164.512(i).

154 45 C.F.R. §§ 164.524 [self], 164.508 [others].

155 E.g., Fla Stat. § 395.017 [hospitals]; § 455.241 [individual professionals]; Ill. Rev. Stat. ch. 110 §§ 8-2001-8-2004; Annotation, Patient's right to disclosure of his or her own medical records under state freedom of information act, 26 A.L.R. 4th 701; Wallace v. University Hosps. of Cleveland, 84 Ohio L. Abs. 224, 170 N.E.2d 261 (Ct. App. 1960).

156 Pierce v. Penman, 357 Pa. Super. 225, 515 A.2d 948 (1986).

157 Franklin Square Hosp. v. Laubach, 318 Md. 615, 569 A.2d 693 (1990).

158 Lee County v. State Farm Mutual Auto. Ins. Co., 634 So. 2d 250 (Fla. 2d DCA 1994).

159 Person v. Farmers Ins. Group, 52 Cal. App. 4th 813, 61 Cal. Rptr. 2d 30 (2d Dist. 1997).

160 E.g., Pyramid Life Ins. Co. v. Masonic Hosp. Ass'n, 191 F. Supp. 51 (W.D. Okla. 1961).

161 45 C.F.R. § 164.510(b).

162 MacDonald v. Clinger, 84 A.D.2d 482, 446 N.Y.S.2d 801 (4th Dept. 1982).

163 E.g., Iowa Code Ann. § 229.25.

164 Thurman v. Crawford, 652 S.W.2d 240 (Mo. Ct. App. 1983).

165 Byers v. Toyota Motor Manufacturing Ky., Inc., 1998 U.S. App. LEXIS 33155 (6th Cir.) (unpub).

166 45 C.F.R. § 164.524(a)(3).

167 Yaretsky v. Blum, 592 F.2d 65 (2d Cir. 1979), appeal after remand, 629 F.2d 817 (2d Cir. 1980), rev'd, 457 U.S. 991 (1982) [no right to hearing before transfer].

168 Salt Lake Child & Family Therapy Clinic, Inc. v. Frederick, 890 P.2d 1017 (Utah 1995).

169 Cynthia B. v. New Rochelle Hosp. Med. Ctr., 60 N.Y.2d 452, 470 N.Y.S.2d 1221, 458 N.E.2d 363 (1983).

170 Doe v. Stincer, 990 F. Supp. 1427 (S.D. Fla. 1997).

171 45 C.F.R. § 164.502(g).

172 E.g., Gaertner v. State, 385 Mich. 49, 187 N.W.2d 429 (1971).

173 45 C.F.R. § 164.524(a)(3)(iii).

174 Mougiannis v. North Shore-Long Island Jewish Health System (N.Y. Sup Ct. May 2004), as reported in N.Y.L.J., May 19, 2004, 19.

175 45 C.F.R. § 164.502(g)(2),(3).

176 E.g., Leaf v. Iowa Methodist Med. Ctr., 460 N.W.2d 892 (Iowa Ct. App. 1990) [noncustodial parent's access right to minor's medical records].

177 E.g. In the Matter of Marriage of Jones, 983 S.W.2d 377 (Tex. App. 1999) [psychologist must disclose records of treatment of minor to parent]; Attorney ad litem for D.K. v. Parents of D.K., 780 So. 2d 301 (Fla. 4th DCA 2001) [minor may block parent access to mental health records]; S.C. v. Guardian ad litem, 845 So. 2d 953 (Fla. 4th DCA 2003) [guardian ad litem cannot have unlimited access to minor's mental health records]; see also T.L. Cheng et al., Confidentiality in health care, 269 J.A.M.A.

1404 (1993) [survey of adolescent attitudes indicated they would not seek health services to avoid disclosure of certain information]; Council on Scientific Affairs, American Med. Ass'n, Confidential health services for adolescents, 269 J.A.M.A. 1420 (1993) [encouraging increased confidentiality].

178 E.g., H.L. v. Matheson, 450 U.S. 398 (1981) [Utah parental consent requirement for abortions].

179 Mrozinski v. Pogue, 205 Ga. App. 731, 423 S.E.2d 405 (1992).

180 45 C.F.R. § 146.502(f).

181 45 C.F.R. § 146.502(g)(4).

182 45 C.F.R. § 146.512 (f)(4), (g), (h).

183 E.g., Scott v. Henry Ford Hosp., 199 Mich. App. 241, 501 N.W.2d 259 (1993) [only executor may authorize release; wife does not have authority]; In Interest of Roy, 423 Pa. Super. 183, 620 A.2d 1172 (1992) [only executor can authorize release of mental health records]; Annotation, Who may waive privilege of confidential communication to physician by person since deceased, 97 A.L.R. 2d 393.

184 E.g., Gerkin v. Werner, 106 Misc. 2d 643, 434 N.Y.S.2d 607 (Sup. Ct. 1980).

185 E.g., Emmett v. Eastern Dispensary and Casualty Hosp., 130 U.S. App. D.C. 50, 396 F.2d 931 (1967).

186 Metropolitan Life Ins. Co. v. Frenette, [1992] 1 S.C.R. 647.

187 Fanshaw v. Medical Protective Ass'n, 52 Wis. 2d 234, 190 N.W.2d 155 (1971).

188 E.g., In re Grand Jury Subpoena for Medical Records of Curtis Payne, 150 N.H. 436, 839 A.2d 837 (2004); Rost v. State Bd. of Psychology, 659 A.2d 626 (Pa. Commw. 1995) [affirming reprimand of psychologist for complying with subpoena by releasing patient records without consent]; Simms v. Bradach, No. MON-L-393-01 (N.J. Super Ct. Monmouth County Sept. 13, 2002), as discussed in H. Gottlieb, Judge bars use of subpoenas for medical records patient's authorization is required, N.J.L.J. Nov. 4, 2002.

189 Washburn v. Rite Aid Corp., 695 A.2d 495 (R.I. 1997).

190 Kunkel v. Walton, 179 Ill. 2d 519, 689 N.E.2d 1047 (1997).

191 45 C.F.R. § 164.512(e)(1)(ii); E.g., Hutton v. City of Martinez, 219 F.R.D. 164 (N.D. Cal. 2003).

192 E.g., Thomas v. Benedictine Hosp., 296 A.D.2d 781, 745 N.Y.S.2d 606 (3d Dept. 2002) [affirming order rejecting plaintiff's effort to depose hospital officials in malpractice lawsuit concerning physician treatment for leg fracture]; Allen v. Smith, 179 W.Va. 360, 368 S.E.2d 924 (1988) [if not protected by statute of limitations, psychiatrist could have been sued for complying with insufficient subpoena].

193 Doe v. Roe, 190 A.D.2d 463, 599 N.Y.S.2d 350 (4th Dept. 1993).

194 E.g., Rojas v. Ryder Truck Rental, Inc., 641 So. 2d 855 (Fla. 1994); Doelfel v. Trevisani, 644 So. 2d 1359 (Fla. 1994).

195 Ritt v. Ritt, 52 N.J. 177, 244 A.2d 497 (1968).

196 Laurent v. Brelji, 74 Ill. App. 3d 214, 392 N.E.2d 929 (4th Dist. 1979).

197 *People v. Bickham*, 89 Ill. 2d 1, 431 N.E.2d 365 (1982).

198 *Roth v. Saint Elizabeth's Hosp.*, 241 Ill. App. 3d 407, 607 N.E.2d 1356 (5th Dist. appeal denied), 151 Ill. 2d 577, 616 N.E.2d 347 (1993).

199 *United States v. Fesman*, 781 F. Supp. 511 (S.D. Ohio 1991).

200 E.g., *Bristol-Meyers Squibb Co. v. Hancock*, 921 S.W.2d 917 (Tex. Ct. App. 1996) [when surgeon sued breast implant manufacturer for injury to his reputation, income, company denied discovery of medical records of his patients]; *Parkson v. Central Du Page Hosp.*, 105 Ill. App. 3d 850, 435 N.E.2d 140 (1st Dist. 1982).

201 E.g., *St. Lukes Reg. Med. Ctr. v. United States*, 717 F. Supp. 665 (N.D. Iowa 1989) [government entitled to disclosure of physician's medical records by administrative subpoena to investigate Medicaid civil violations]; *Goldberg v. Davis*, 151 Ill. 2d 267, 602 N.E.2d 812 (1992) [professional discipline]; *Dr. K v. State Bd. of Physician Quality Assurance*, 98 Md. App. 103, 632 A.2d 453, cert. denied, 513 U.S. 817 (1994) [professional discipline].

202 E.g., *Amente v. Newman*, 653 So. 2d 1030 (Fla. 1995); *Todd v. South Jersey Hosp. Sys.*, 152 F.R.D. 676 (D. N.J. 1993); *Terre Haute Reg. Hosp. v. Trueblood*, 600 N.E.2d 1358 (Ind. 1992); *Community Hosp. Ass'n v. District Court*, 194 Colo. 98, 570 P.2d 243 (1977); State ex rel. *Lester E. Cox Med. Ctr. v. Keet*, 678 S.W.2d 813 (Mo. 1984) (en banc).

203 E.g., *Buford v. Howe*, 10 F.3d 1184 (5th Cir. 1994); *Glassman v. St. Joseph Hosp.*, 259 Ill. App. 3d 730, 631 N.E.2d 1186 (1st Dist. 1994); *Ekstrom v. Temple*, 197 Ill. App. 3d 120, 553 N.E.2d 424 (2d Dist. 1990).

204 People ex rel. *Dep't of Prof'l Regulation v. Manos*, 202 Ill. 2d 563, 578 (Ill. 2002).

205 *Schechet v. Kesten*, 372 Mich. 346, 126 N.W.2d 718 (1964); *Dorris v. Detroit Osteopathic Hosp. Corp.*, 559 N.W.2d 76 (Mich. Ct. App. 1996) [affirming denial of disclosure of name of nonparty patient who may have witnessed patient's refusal of drug]; accord *Gunn v. Sound Shore Med. Ctr.*, 5 A.D.3d 435, 772 N.Y.S.2d 714 (2d Dept. 2004) [reject release of log of patients in rehab center when accident happened].

206 *Kinsella v. NYT Television*, 382 N.J. Super. 102, 110 (N.J. Super. 2005).

207 E.g., *City of Edmund v. Parr*, 587 P.2d 56 (Okla. 1978); *Jenkins v. Wu*, 102 Ill. 2d 468, 468 N.E.2d 1162 (1984); but see *Southwest Commun. Health Servs. v. Smith*, 107 N.M. 196, 755 P.2d 40 (1988) [law upheld, but court may ignore law when records sufficiently needed in litigation].

208 *Dir. of Health Affairs Policy Planning v. Freedom of Info. Comm'n*, 293 Conn. 164 (Conn. 2009).

209 *Young v. King*, 136 N.J. Super. 127, 344 A.2d 792 (Law Div. 1975).

210 *Brandon Reg'l Hosp. v. Murray*, 957 So. 2d 590, 591 (Fla. 2007).

211 Id.

212 *Hosp. Auth. v. Meeks*, 285 Ga. 521 (Ga. 2009).

213 State ex rel. *Shroades v. Henry*, 187 W.Va. 723, 421 S.E.2d 264 (1992).

214 E.g., *Carr v. Howard*, 426 Mass. 514, 689 N.E.2d 1304 (1998) [reports for peer review committee confidential, cannot be provided to trial judge for in camera review]; Application to Quash a Grand Jury Subpoena, 239 A.D.2d 412, 657 N.Y.S.2d 747 (2d Dept. 1997) [quashing grand jury subpoena of hospital's quality assurance records].

215 Ex parte Fairfield Nursing & Rehab. Ctr., L.L.C., 22 So. 3d 445, 450 (Ala. 2009).

216 *Warrick v. Giron*, 290 N.W.2d 166 (Minn. 1980).

217 E.g., *Cedars-Sinai Med. Ctr. v. Superior Court*, 12 Cal. App. 4th 579, 16 Cal. Rptr. 2d 253 (2d Dist. 1993).

218 *Huntsman v. Aultman Hosp.*, 160 Ohio App. 3d 196, 2005 Ohio 1482, 826 N.E.2d 384.

219 E.g., *Ashokan v. Department of Ins.*, 109 Nev. 662, 856 P.2d 244 (1993).

220 E.g., Fla. Stat. §§ 395.0191–395.0193, 766.101; *Young v. Saldanha*, 189 W.Va. 330, 431 S.E.2d 669 (1993) [physician's use of peer review materials in suit against hospital concerning clinical privileges did not waive evidentiary privilege, so patient could not use materials in malpractice suit against physician].

221 E.g., *St. Elizabeth's Hosp. v. State Bd. of Prof. Med. Conduct*, 174 A.D.2d 225, 579 N.Y.S.2d 457 (3d Dept. 1992).

222 *Adams v. St. Francis Reg. Med. Ctr.*, 264 Kan. 144, 955 P.2d 1169 (1998).

223 42 U.S.C. § 11111(a)(1).

224 Id. at § 11101(5).

225 Id. at § 11101; see also *Moore v. Williamsburg Reg'l Hosp.*, 560 F.3d 166, 171 (4th Cir. S.C. 2009) (discussing the purpose of HCQIA).

226 42 U.S.C. § 11151(9).

227 Id. at § 11112(a).

228 http://www.iom.edu/~/media/Files/Report%20Files/1999/To-Err-is-Human/To%20Err%20is%20Human%201999%20%20report%20brief.pdf

229 http://www.ahrq.gov/qual/psoact.htm

230 http://www.pso.ahrq.gov/listing/alphalist.htm

231 45 C.F.R. §§ 164.512, 164.103 ["required by law"].

232 E.g., Fla. Stat. §§ 382.16, 382.081.

233 E.g., Fla. Stat. § 381.231 [communicable diseases], § 384.25 [venereal diseases].

234 *Derrick v. Ontario Comm. Hosp.*, 47 Cal. App. 3d 145, 120 Cal. Rptr. 566 (4th Dist. 1975).

235 State ex rel. *Callahan v. Kinder*, 879 S.W.2d 677 (Mo. Ct. App. 1994).

236 E.g., Fla. Stat. § 415.504; L.S. Wissow, Current concepts: Child abuse and neglect, 332 N. Eng. J. Med. 1425 (1995).

237 45 C.F.R. § 164.512(b)(1)(ii).

238 E.g., Wis. Stat. § 48.981(2)(a).

239 See A. Goldstein, Hospital for priests not required to report all abuse, WASH. POST, June 30, 2002, C5 [Maryland AG opinion, provider not required to report abuse outside of state].

240 E.g., *O'Heron v. Blaney,* 276 Ga. 871, 583 S.E.2d 834 (2003); *Meyer v. Lashley,* 44 P.2d 553 (Okla. 2002); *Casbohm v. Metrohealth Med. Ctr.,* 746 N.E.2d 661 (Ohio. App. 2000); *Martinez v. Mafchir,* 35 F.3d 1486 (10th Cir. 1994) [social worker protected]; see also *People v. Wood,* 447 Mich. 80, 523 N.W.2d 477 (1994) [social worker could contact police to obtain assistance in investigating possible neglect]; *Bryant-Bruce v. Vanderbilt Univ. Inc.,* 974 F. Supp. 1127. (M.D. Tenn. 1997) [immunity only for report within scope of state duty to report; deny dismissal for other aspects of report]; *Bol v. Cole,* 561 N.W.2d 143 (Minn. 1997) [no immunity for copy of report given to patient's mother; only qualified privilege to release to mother to protect child who cannot otherwise protect self].

241 E.g., *Gladson v. State,* 258 Ga. 885, 376 S.E.2d 362 (1989); Doctor faces penalty for failing to report child abuse, AP, Nov. 8, 2002 [Iowa MD fined $5,000 in settlement with licensing board]; Prosecutors drop charges against doctors accused of failing to report child abuse, AP, Feb. 11, 2004 [Mich.].

242 E.g., IOWA CODE ANN. § 232.75(2); *Stecker v. First Commercial Trust Co.,* 962 S.W.2d 792 (Ark. 1998); *Landeros v. Flood,* 17 Cal. 3d 399, 131 Cal. Rptr. 69, 551 P.2d 389 (1976); contra, *Vance v. T.R.C.,* 229 Ga. App. 608. 494 S.E.2d 714 (1997) [statute requiring child abuse report did not create private cause of action against physician for failure to report]; Annotation, Validity, construction, and application of state statute requiring doctor or other person to report child abuse, 73 A.L.R. 4TH 782; Jury reaches $2 million verdict in injuries to abused infant, AP, Apr. 29, 2002 [Missouri physician, day care center liable]; but see *Cuyler v. United States,* 362 F.3d 949 (7th Cir. 2004) [no implied duty of rescue in Ill. child abuse statute, so no civil liability].

243 Missouri reporting law for healthcare workers is unconstitutional, AP, Sept. 11, 2003; Missouri Supreme Court to hear arguments in nurse appeal, AP, Apr. 30, 2004.

244 E.g., *People v. Stockton Pregnancy Control Med. Clinic,* 203 Cal. App. 3d 225, 249 Cal. Rptr. 762 (3d Dist. 1988) [must report sexual conduct of minors under age 14 if with person of disparate age]; *Planned Parenthood Affiliates v. Van de Camp,* 181 Cal. App. 3d 245, 226 Cal. Rptr. 361 (1st Dist. 1986) [not required to report all sexual activity of minors under age 14]; Doctor seeks special probation, AP, Dec. 12, 2002 [two-year probation for Conn. MD accused of failing to report pregnancy of 10-year-old; J. Hanna, Kline: Doctors must report youngsters' pregnancies, AP, June 18, 2002 [Kansas AG opinion]; R. Hegeman, Kansas judge says doctors cannot be forced to report underage sex, AP, July 26, 2004; see also WIS. STAT. § 48.981(2m) [providers not required to report some sexual activities of minors].

245 E.g., FLA STAT. § 415.103; M.S. Lachs & K. Pillemer, Current concepts: Abuse and neglect of elderly persons, 332 N. ENG. J. MED. 437 (1995) [42 states required reporting in 1991].

246 E.g., WIS. STAT. § 46.90 [elder abuse].

247 45 C.F.R. § 164.512(c).

248 S. Stapleton, Confidentiality is key in protecting patients, AM. MED. NEWS, July 14, 1997, 3 [Am. Med. Ass'n opposes reporting domestic violence]; A. Hyman et al., Laws mandating reporting of domestic violence: Do they promote patient well-being? 273 J.A.M.A. 1781 (1995) [questioning helpfulness where there are inadequate responses to reports]; see also S. Stapleton, Plans ask doctors to address domestic violence, AM. MED. NEWS, Dec. 21, 1998, 28 [internal reporting within managed care].

249 See D. Hancock, Hospital's inaction delayed arrest, MIAMI (FL) HERALD, Jan. 24, 1996, 6B [no notice to authorities of gunshot victim as required, gave clothing (potential evidence) to family].

250 N.Y. PENAL LAW § 265.25.

251 IOWA CODE ANN. § 147.111.

252 In the Matter of Grand Jury Investigation in New York County, 98 N.Y.2d 525, 779 N.E.2d 173, 749 N.Y.S.2d 462 (2002); but see *State v. Baptist Mem. Hosp.,* 726 So. 2d 554 (Miss. 1998) [state can subpoena records of all patients treated for lacerations during a specified time period as part of a homicide investigation, where the law requires reporting knifings which the court broadly interpreted to include the cases sought by the subpoena].

253 See American Medical Association wants doctors more involved with older drivers, AP Sept. 10, 2003; J.E. Allen, Medicine: Drivers not telling doctors of seizures: Some report concealing episodes because they don't want to lose their licenses, a survey finds, L.A. TIMES, Apr. 7, 2003, 3 [6 states require reports of seizures]; WIS. STAT. § 146.82(3)(a) [permissive]; see also Edina hospital cited for allowing drugged patient drive, AP Aug. 5, 2003 [MN hospital given three citations]; M. Raffaele, Six-pack-a-day drinker loses license, AP, July 13, 2004 [challenge to loss after MD report].

254 E.g., FLA. ADMIN. CODE §§ 10D-91.425, 10D-91.426, 10D-91.428 [radiation incidents].

255 21 C.F.R. § 606.170(b).

256 21 C.F.R. § 812.150(b).

257 21 U.S.C. § 360, 21 C.F.R. § 803.

258 E.g., *Beth Israel Hosp. Ass'n v. Board of Registration in Med.,* 401 Mass. 172, 515 N.E.2d 574 (1987).

259 *Choe v. Axelrod,* 141 A.D.2d 235, 534 N.Y.S.2d 739 (3d Dept. 1988).

260 *Whalen v. Roe,* 429 U.S. 589 (1977).

261 E.g., 42 U.S.C. § 300ff-132.

262 See Annotation, Liability of doctor or other health practitioner to third party contracting contagious disease from doctor's patient, 3 A.L.R. 5TH 370.

263 *Derrick v. Ontario Commun. Hosp.,* 47 Cal. App. 3d 154, 120 Cal Rptr. 566 (4th Dist. 1975).

264 *Phillips v. Oconee Mem. Hosp.,* 290 S.C. 192, 348 S.E.2d 836 (1986).

265 *Tarasoff v. Regents of Univ. of Cal.,* 17 Cal. 3d 425, 131 Cal. Rptr. 14, 551 P.2d 334 (1976).

266 *Thompson v. County of Alameda,* 27 Cal. 3d 741, 167 Cal. Rptr. 70, 614 P.2d 728 (1980).

267 E.g., *Thornburg v. Long*, 178 N.C. 589, 101 S.E. 99 (1919); see also *Gross v. Allen*, 22 Cal. App. 4th 354, 27 Cal. Rptr. 2d 429 (2d Dist. 1994) [original psychiatrists had duty to tell subsequent attending psychiatrist of patient's prior suicide attempts; subsequent psychiatrist called to obtain history].

268 E.g., *Watts v. Cumberland County Hosp. Sys.*, 75 N.C. App. 1, 330 S.E.2d

269 45 C.F.R. § 164.512(b).

270 45 C.F.R. § 164.512(d).

271 45 C.F.R. § 164.512(e).

272 45 C.F.R. § 164.512(f).

273 45 C.F.R. § 164.512(h).

274 45 C.F.R. § 164.512(i).

275 45 C.F.R. § 164.512(j).

276 45 C.F.R. § 164.512(k).

277 45 C.F.R. §§ 164.512(a)(1) [named patient], 164.512(f)(2) [suspect, fugitive, material witness, missing person]; 164.512(f)(3) [victim].

278 See 45 C.F.R. § 512(k)(5); *Johnson v. West Va. Univ. Hosps., Inc.*, 186 W.Va. 648, 413 S.E.2d 889 (1991) [liability for failure to warn hospital security guard of HIV status of patient before asking him to assist in restraint of patient].

279 E.g., M. Stolz, Politician's drug records protected; Judge says police lacked warrant to get evidence from pharmacy, Plain Dealer, Mar. 15, 2002, B3 [Ohio trial court threw out records in prosecution for allegedly lying to obtain pain drugs].

280 E.g., *Ferguson v. City of Charleston*, 532 U.S. 67 (2001) [performing urine tests at request of law enforcement to obtain evidence of cocaine use by maternity patients for law enforcement purposes was unreasonable search violating Fourth Amendment].

281 E.g., *Comm. v. Shaw*, 564 Pa. 617, 770 A.2d 295 (2001) [clinical blood test results obtained by police without warrant not admissible]; *State v. Dyal*, 97 N.J. 229, 478 A.2d 390 (1984) [court-issued subpoena required when police seek to obtain hospital blood test]; contra, *People v. Ernst*, 311 Ill. App. 3d 672, 725 N.E.2d 59 (2d Dist. 2000) [hospital may disclose blood alcohol results to police without court order]; *Hannoy v. State*, 793 N.E.2d 1109 (Ind. App. 2003) [clinical blood alcohol results may be released to police without court order]; but see *State v. Schreiber*, 122 N.J. 579, 585 A.2d 945 (1991) [doctor initiated disclosure of blood test result admissible]; *Tapp v. State*, 108 S.W.3d 459 (Tex. App. 2003) [upholding obtaining clinical blood test results with a grand jury subpoena].

282 E.g., *People v. Gomez*, 147 Misc. 2d 704, 556 N.Y.S.2d 961 (Sup. Ct. 1990) [police witness surgical removal of bags from stomach].

283 *State v. Thompson*, 585 N.W.2d 905 (Wis. App. 1998).

284 E.g., *Comm. v. Johnson*, 556 Pa. 216, 727 A.2d 1089 (1999) [no reasonable expectation of privacy in bullet removed for medical reasons, so no violation to give to police without warrant]; *State v. Cowan*, 46 S.W.2d 227 (Tenn. Crim. App. 2000) [no reasonable expectation of privacy in removed bullet, so admissible even though obtained from hospital without warrant].

285 45 C.F.R. § 164.512(k)(2),(3).

286 45 C.F.R. §§ 164.310(c), 164.502(a)(2)(ii).

287 45 C.F.R. § 164.512(d).

288 E.g., Iowa Code Ann. § 85.27.

289 E.g., *Acosta v. Cary*, 365 So. 2d 4 (La. Ct. App. 1978).

290 *Morris v. Consolidation Coal Co.*, 191 W.Va. 426, 446 S.E.2d 648 (1994).

291 45 C.F.R. § 164.512(l).

292 5 U.S.C. § 552.

293 5 U.S.C. § 552a; *Doe v. Stephens*, 271 U.S. App. D.C. 230, 851 F.2d 1457 (1988) [effect of Privacy Act on grand jury subpoena of VA medical records]; *Williams v. Department of Veterans Affairs*, 879 F. Supp. 578 (E.D. Va. 1995) [Privacy Act is exclusive remedy for wrongful disclosure of medical information by VA].

294 E.g., Iowa Code Ann. § 22.7; *Head v. Colloton*, 331 N.W.2d 870 (Iowa 1983).

295 *Eugene Cervi & Co. v. Russell*, 184 Colo. 282, 519 P.2d 1189 (1974).

296 *Head v. Colloton*, 331 N.W.2d 870 (Iowa 1983).

297 *Wooster Republican Printing Co. v. City of Wooster*, 56 Ohio St. 2d 126, 383 N.E.2d 124 (1978).

298 E.g., *Oklahoma Disability Law Ctr. v. Dillon Family & Youth Servs.*, 879 F. Supp. 1110 (D. Okla. 1995) [plaintiff entitled to discovery of treatment records of its clients, state law authorizing facility to require court order superseded by federal Protection and Advocacy of Mentally Ill Individuals Act].

299 18 U.S.C. § 2511(d).

300 *Estate of Berthiaume v. Pratt*, 365 A.2d 792 (Me. 1976); see Annotation, Taking unauthorized photographs as invasion of privacy, 86 A.L.R. 3d 374.

301 *Anderson v. Strong Mem. Hosp.*, 140 Misc. 2d 770, 531 N.Y.S.2d 735 (Sup. Ct. 1988), aff'd, 151 A.D.2d 1033, 542 N.Y.S.2d 96 (4th Dept. 1989).

302 E.g., *Stubbs v. North Mem. Med. Ctr.*, 448 N.W.2d 78 (Minn. Ct. App. 1989) [publication in promotional, educational materials of before, after photographs of facial cosmetic surgery without patient consent may constitute breach of express warranty of silence arising from physician-patient relationship]; *Feeney v. Young*, 191 A.D. 501, 181 N.Y.S. 481 (1st Dept. 920) [public showing of a film of a caesarean section delivery]; *Vassiliades v. Garfinkels*, 492 A.2d 580 (D.C. 1985) [public use of before, after photos of cosmetic surgery in department store, on television]; see Annotation, Invasion of privacy by use of plaintiff's name or likeness in advertising, 23 A.L.R. 3d 865.

303 *In re Simmons*, 112 A.D.2d 806, 492 N.Y.S.2d 308 (4th Dept. 1985); but see *North Broward Hosp. Dist. v. ABC*, No. 86-026514 (Fla. Cir. Ct. Broward County Oct. 20, 1986) [hospital cannot prohibit media access to comatose patient when guardian consents].

304 R.J. Peach, Court overrides hospital's ban on photographs in intensive care unit, Legal Intelligencer, Dec. 27, 2000, 6.

305 E.g., Jury acquits reporter of trespassing charge, AP Dec. 23, 2003 [N.C. reporter entered assisted living center with assistance of former staff member and videotaped sleeping residents].

306 *Shulman v. Group W Productions*, 18 Cal. 4th 200, 74 Cal. Rptr. 2d 843, 955 P.2d 469 (1998).

307 E.g., Nurse accused of torturing brain-damaged child, AP Oct. 3, 2003 [use of film from surveillance cameras in WA home installed by grandmother]; Mother accused of contaminating infant daughter's IV, AP, Jan. 15, 2004 [Ind. woman videotaped injecting fecal matter into daughter's IV tube]; *Kinsella v. Welch*, 2003 N.J. Super. LEXIS 253 (App. Div.) [under newsperson privilege media not required to produce video of treatment in hospital, but must produce any portions that will be used at trial].

308 Judge: Media permitted to broadcast video of woman in coma, AP, Oct. 2, 2002.

309 Lawsuit: Woman claims doctor branded her during surgery, AP, Jan. 24, 2003.

310 2011 JC CAMH, RI.01.03.01.

311 Bush promotes technology, UPI, Apr. 26, 2004.

312 See *Schmidt v. U.S. Dep't Of Veterans Affairs*, 218 F.R.D. 619 (E.D. Wis. 2003).

313 Described in http://www.phdsc.org/standards/fse.asp (accessed Mar. 4, 2012).

314 The office website is http://healthit.hhs.gov/portal/server.pt/community/healthit_hhs_gov__home/1204 (accessed Mar. 4, 2012).

315 M. Freudenheim, Many hospitals resist computerized patient care, N.Y. TIMES, Apr. 6, 2004, C1; R. Koppel et al., Role of computerized physician order entry systems in facilitating medication errors, J.A.M.A., Mar. 9, 2005, 1197.

316 See S. Lohr, Healthcare technology is a promise unfinanced, N.Y. TIMES, Dec. 3, 2004, C5; J. Morrissey, It's more than just the purchase; make clear the commitments that it will trigger, MOD. HEALTHCARE, July 12, 2004, 30.

317 E.g., *Doe v. Medlantic Health Care Group*, 814 A.2d 939 (D.C. App. 2003) [hospital liable under D.C. law for staff member's dissemination of HIV status after unauthorized lookup]; *Doe v. Dartmouth-Hitchcock Med. Ctr.*, 2001 U.S. Dist. LEXIS 10704 (D.N.H.) [hospital not liable under federal law for MD lookup]; J. Mandak, Researcher sentenced in Wynette case, AP Online, Dec. 1, 2000 [using former physician's password, former research assistant accessed computerized hospital records of late country singer Tammy Wynette and sold them to tabloids; sentenced to six months, fined amount received from tabloids]; *Arbster v. Unemployment Comp. Bd. of Rev.*, 690 A.2d 805 (Pa. Commw. 1997) [nurse fired for lookup of computer records of her family denied unemployment compensation]; see also *Schmidt v. U.S. Dep't of Veterans Affairs*, 218 F.R.D. 619 (E.D. Wis. 2003) [challenge to access to employee social security numbers in VA hospital computerized medical record; description of steps VA had taken to restrict, trace lookups].

318 Electronic Signatures in Global and National Consumer Act, Pub. No. L. 106-229, 114 Stat, 464 (2000), codified in part at 15 U.S. §§ 7001 et seq.

319 E.g., Second doctor sues hospital over Pap smear tests, AP, Jan. 23, 2004 [accusation of misuse of electronic signatures]; Feds find no significant problems with Magee Pap smears, AP, Apr. 13, 2004.

320 *Whalen v. Roe*, 429 U.S. 589 (1977); see also Letcher woman convicted on drug fraud charges, AP, Apr. 4, 2001 [use of KY computerized prescription tracking system to achieve conviction].

321 E.g., 15 U.S.C. § 7001; *United States v. Fujii*, 301 F.3d 535 (7th Cir. 2002) [admissibility of printouts in federal court].

322 See http://www.nlm.nih.gov/research/umls/Snomed/snomed_faq.html (accessed Mar. 4, 2012).

323 See L. Stevens, Virtually there, AM. MED. NEWS, Dec. 21, 1998, 24; B. Kane & D.Z. Sands, Guidelines for the clinical use of electronic mail with patients, 5 J. AM. MED. INFORMATICS ASS'N 104 (1998) [http://jamia.bmj.com/content/5/1/104.full.pdf+html; accessed Mar. 4, 2012]; S.M. Borowitz & J.C. Wyatt, The origin, content, and workload of e-mail consultations, J.A.M.A., Oct. 21, 1998, 1321; A.R. Spielberg, On call and online: Sociohistorical, legal, and ethical implications of e-mail for the patient physician relationship, J.A.M.A., Oct. 21, 1998, 1353; G. Baldwin, Doctor benefits from e-mail efficiency with patients, AM. MED. NEWS, Dec. 21, 1998, 24.

324 *Walgreen Co. v. Wisconsin Pharmacy Examining Bd.*, 217 Wis. 2d 290, 577 N.W.2d 387, 1998 Wisc. App. LEXIS 201 (Unpub).

325 See Online consultations slow to take off, AM. MED. NEWS, Apr. 12, 2004, 21 [consumers say they want e-mail, but unwilling to pay more than $10].

326 E.g., L. Kowalczyk, The doctor will e-you now: Insurers to pay doctors to answer questions over Web, BOSTON GLOBE, May 24, 2004, A1.

327 E.g., A. Michaels & D. Wells, HealthSouth investigators reveal damning new e-mail, FINANCIAL TIMES (London), July 11, 2003, 13; J. Sarche, Beware of e-mail, text messages, WIS. ST. J., June 7, 2004, A3.

328 E.g., *United States v. Councilman*, 2004 U.S. App. LEXIS 13352 (1st Cir.).

329 E.g., M.A. Nusbaum, New kind of snooping arrives at the office, N.Y. TIMES, July 13, 2003, 12BU.

330 E.g., Georgia man accused of sending Internet threat to hospital, AP, Mar. 6, 2003.

331 E.g., J. Wells, Wrong MDs got patient records; psychiatric privacy violated, SAN FRANCISCO CHRONICLE, Dec. 30, 2000, A13; M.W. Salganik, Health data on 858 patients mistakenly e-mailed to others; medical information was among messages sent out by Kaiser Health Care, BALTIMORE SUN, Aug. 10, 2000, 1C.

332 E.g., Hacker steals files on patients from UW, SEATTLE TIMES, Dec. 9, 2000, B1 [hacker stole files on 4,700 patients].

333 See S. Bakerand & M. Shenk, A patch in time saves nine: Liability risks for unpatched software, CORP. COUNSELLOR, Apr. 5, 2004, 3.

334 E.g., M. Lerner & J. Marcotty, Web posting has health and university officials scrambling; mental health records of children from 20 families were mistakenly put onto the Internet, STAR TRIBUNE (Minneapolis, MN), Nov. 8, 2001, 1B; C. Pillar, Web mishap: Kids' psychological files posted, L.A. TIMES, Nov. 7, 2001, A1.

335 *Planned Parenthood v. American Coalition of Life Activists,* 41 F. Supp. 2d 1130 (D. Or. 1999), rev'd, 244 F.3d 1007 (9th Cir. 2001), rev'd, 290 F.3d 1058 (9th Cir. 2002) (en banc) [reinstating district court injunction and verdict against defendants], cert. denied, 123 S. Ct. 2637 (U.S. 2003), on remand, 300 F. Supp. 2d 1055 (D. Ore. 2004) [jury award of punitive damages affirmed].

336 T. Hillig & J. Mannies, Woman sues over posting of abortion details; her records from Granite City hospital were put on website; hospital, protesters are defendants, St. Louis Post-Dispatch, July 3, 2001, A1; J. Mannies, Abortion foes are ordered to take woman's records, photo off Web; patient had complications at clinic in Granite City, St. Louis Post-Dispatch, July 11, 2001, B1; Judge keeps woman's records off net, AP Online, Aug. 23, 2001.

337 A. Barnard, Facing criticism cosmetic surgeon sues over postings by a former patient, Boston Globe, Sept. 24, 2002, B1; see also M. Ko, Judge limits police data online; website operators must remove officers' Social Security numbers, Seattle Times, May 11, 2001, B; A. Liptak, Dispute simmers over website posting personal data on police, N.Y. Times, July 12, 2003, A1.

338 J. Mandak, Judge orders attorneys to shut down hospital lawsuit website, AP, Dec. 23, 2003 [E.D. Pa. judge ordered closing site recruiting for class action suit against hospital]; Law firms, hospital agree.

Information Management

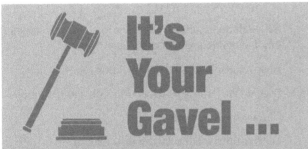

FATAL HANDWRITING MIX-UP

Forty-two-year-old Vasquez died as a result of a handwriting mix-up on the medication prescribed for his heart. Vasquez had been given a prescription for 20 mg of Isordil to be taken four times per day. The pharmacist misread the physician's handwriting and filled the prescription with Plendil, a drug for high blood pressure, which is usually taken at no more than 10 mg per day. As a result, Vasquez was given the wrong medication at eight times the recommended dosage. He died 2 weeks later from an apparent heart attack. The family filed a lawsuit.[1]

WHAT IS YOUR VERDICT?

Reducing Medical Errors

To significantly reduce the tens of thousands of deaths and injuries caused by medical errors every year, health care organizations must adopt information technology systems that are capable of collecting and sharing essential health information on patients and their care, says a new report by the Institute of Medicine of the National Academies. These systems should operate seamlessly as part of a national network of health information that is accessible by all health care organizations and that includes electronic records of patients' care, secure platforms for the exchange of information among providers and patients, and data standards that will make health information uniform and understandable to all, said the committee that wrote the report.

—Institute of Medicine, "Reducing Medical Errors Requires National Computerized Information Systems; Data Standards Are Crucial to Improving Patient Safety," News, November 20, 2003; http://www8.nationalacademies.org/onpinews/ newsitem.aspx?RecordID=10863.

The effective and efficient delivery of patient care requires that an organization determine its information needs. Organizations that do not centralize their information needs will often suffer scattered databases, which may result in such problems as duplication of data gathering, inconsistent reports, and inefficiencies in the use of economic resources.

As the principal means of communication between healthcare professionals in matters relating to patient care, the medical record primarily provides documentation of a patient's illness, symptoms, diagnosis, and treatment and is used as a planning tool for patient care. Practitioners also use medical records to document communication;

assist in protecting the legal interests of the patient, the organization, and the practitioner; provide a database for use in statistical reporting, continuing education, and research; and provide information necessary for third-party billing and regulatory agencies. Healthcare organizations are required to maintain a medical record for each patient in accordance with accepted professional standards and practices.

Nurses tend to access the medical record more often than other healthcare professionals, simply because of the greater amount of time spent caring for patients. Because of the job description, the nurse monitors the patient's illness, response to medication, display of pain and discomfort, and general condition. The patient's care, as well as the nurse's observations, should be recorded on a regular basis. A nurse who has doubt as to the appropriateness of a particular order should verify with the physician the intent of the prescribed order.

Licensure rules and regulations contained in state statutes generally describe the requirements and standards for the maintenance, handling, signing, filing, and retention of medical records. Failure to maintain a complete and accurate medical record reflecting the treatment rendered may affect the ability of an organization and/or physician to obtain third-party reimbursement (e.g., from Medicare, Medicaid, or private insurance carriers). Under federal and state laws, the medical record must reflect accurately the treatment for which the organization or physician seeks payment. Thus, the medical record is important to the organization for medical, legal, and financial reasons.

State laws often contain provisions mandating that organizations maintain a complete medical record for each patient that contains all pertinent information regarding the daily care and treatment of that patient. Medical records must be complete, accurate, current, readily accessible, and systematically organized. This chapter reviews the legal aspects of patient and physician information, communications, and finances.

MANAGING INFORMATION

 iPhone Provides Vital Link to Medical Records

Saving lives means making fast, informed decisions. And at Toronto's Mount Sinai Hospital, iPhone instantly delivers the information that physicians need to make critical treatment decisions. The hospital recently developed VitalHub, an in-house built iPhone app that gives physicians secure, remote access to patient records, test results, vital statistics, and medical literature from its vast internal data network. Using VitalHub on iPhone

allows Mount Sinai's clinicians to respond more rapidly to patient needs wherever and whenever they arise.

— Apple, "iPhone Provides Vital Link to Medical Records," http://www.apple.com/iphone/business/ profiles/mt-sinai/?sr=hotnews.rss.

All organizations, regardless of mission or size, develop and maintain information management systems, which often include financial, medical, and human resource data. Information management is a process intended to facilitate the flow of information within and between departments and caregivers. An information management plan should:

- Determine customer needs, both internal and external (e.g., third-party payers)

- Set goals and establish priorities (e.g., the development of an integrated patient care record)

- Improve accuracy of data collection

- Provide uniformity of data collection and definitions

- Limit duplication of entries

- Deliver timely and accurate information

- Provide easy access to information

- Maintain security and confidentiality of information

- Enhance patient care activities

- Improve collaboration across the organization through information sharing

- Establish disaster plans for the recovery of information

- Orient and train staff on the information management system

- Provide an annual review of the information plan to include its scope, organization, objectives, and effectiveness

CONTENTS OF MEDICAL RECORDS

Because the medical record fulfills many crucial roles within a healthcare organization, practitioners must strive to fulfill all requirements to maintain the integrity and accuracy of the records. The inpatient medical record includes:

- The admission record, which describes pertinent data regarding the patient's age, address, reason for admission, Social Security number, marital status, religion, health insurance, and other information necessary to meet both federal and state requirements

- Consent and authorization for treatment forms allowing the healthcare facility to perform various procedures, such as routine diagnostic testing

- Advance directives

- Medical history and physical examination, including diagnosis and findings that support the diagnosis

- Patient screenings and assessments (e.g., nursing, functional, nutritional, social, and discharge planning)

- Treatment plan

- Physicians' orders

- Progress notes

- Nursing notes (where an integrated record exists, nursing notes are often placed in the progress notes, along with the notes of other disciplines)

- Diagnostic reports (e.g., laboratory and imaging)

- Consultation reports

- Vital signs charts

- Fluid intake and output charts

- Pain management records

- Anesthesia assessment

- Operative reports

- Medication administration records

- Discharge planning/social service notes and reports

- Patient education

- Discharge summaries

OWNERSHIP AND RELEASE OF MEDICAL RECORDS

Healthcare providers who handle medical records must fully understand the related issues of ownership and privacy. Medical records are the property of the provider of care and are maintained for the benefit of the patient. Ownership resides with the organization or professional rendering treatment. Although medical records typically have been protected from public scrutiny by a general practice of nondisclosure, this practice has been waived under a limited number of specifically controlled situations. Some jurisdictions recognize that individuals have a right to privacy and to be protected from the mass dissemination of information pertaining to their personal or private affairs. The right of

privacy generally includes the right to be kept out of the public spotlight. The Privacy Act of 1974 was enacted to safeguard individual privacy from the misuse of federal records and to give individuals access to records concerning themselves that are maintained by federal agencies.

Privacy Act of 1974

 Hospital Workers Punished for Peeking at Clooney File

George Clooney and his companion got top billing when they were treated at a New Jersey hospital after a motorcycle accident last month. But while some nurses clamored to see the celebrity patients, other staff members were busy prying into the couple's medical records, hospital officials said yesterday.

That curiosity proved to be costly. After an internal investigation, the hospital, Palisades Medical Center in North Bergen, has suspended 27 employees for a month without pay for violating a federal law on patient confidentiality.

—Bruce Lambert and Nate Schweber, "Hospital Workers Punished for Peeking at Clooney File," The New York Times, October 10, 2007; http://www.nytimes.com/2007/10/10/ nyregion/10clooney.html?_r=1.

The Privacy Act of 1974, codified at 5 U.S.C. 552, was enacted to safeguard individual privacy from the misuse of federal records, to give individuals access to records concerning themselves that are maintained by federal agencies, and to establish a Privacy Protection Safety Commission. Section 2 of the Privacy Act reads as follows:

[a] The Congress finds that (1) the privacy of an individual is directly affected by the collection, maintenance, use, and dissemination of personal information by Federal agencies; (2) the increasing use of computers and sophisticated information technology, while essential to the efficient operations of the Government, has greatly magnified the harm to individual privacy that can occur from any collection, maintenance, use, or dissemination of personal information; (3) the opportunities for an individual to secure employment, insurance, and credit, and his right to due process, and other legal protections are

endangered by the misuse of certain information systems; (4) the right to privacy is a personal and fundamental right protected by the Constitution of the United States; and (5) in order to protect the privacy of individuals identified in information systems maintained by Federal agencies, it is necessary and proper for the Congress to regulate the collection, maintenance, use, and dissemination of information by such agencies. [b] The purpose of this Act is to provide certain safeguards for an individual against an invasion of personal privacy by requiring Federal agencies, except as otherwise provided by law, to (1) permit an individual to determine what records pertaining to him are collected, maintained, used, or disseminated by such agencies; (2) permit an individual to prevent records pertaining to him obtained by such agencies for a particular purpose from being used or made available for another purpose without his consent; (3) permit an individual to gain access to information pertaining to him in Federal agency records, to have a copy made of all or any portion thereof, and to correct or amend such records; (4) collect, maintain, use, or disseminate any record of identifiable personal information in a manner that assures that such action is for a necessary and lawful purpose, that the information is current and accurate for its intended use, and that adequate safeguards are provided to prevent misuse of such information. . . .

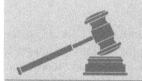

RELEASE OF CONFIDENTIAL INFORMATION

Citation: Proenza Sanfiel v. Department of Health, 749 So. 2d 525 (Fla. App. 1999)

Facts

Sanfiel, a psychiatric nurse, had his professional license suspended for 5 years after he intentionally disclosed confidential patient information to the news media. Sanfiel testified that he knew the information he possessed was confidential and that he understood the danger in disclosing psychiatric records to unauthorized persons. He also knew that a nurse could be disciplined for disclosing such

information, yet he intentionally released information to the news media. The state board of nursing suspended Sanfiel's nursing license and placed him on probation for 5 years for disclosing confidential patient information.

Issue

Was the state board of nursing authorized to suspend Sanfiel's license because of his disclosure of information to the news media?

Holding

Sanfiel's professional license was properly suspended for a 5-year period after he intentionally disclosed confidential patient information to the news media.

Reason

Sanfiel obtained a computer, which was previously owned by Charter Behavioral Health System psychiatric hospital in Orlando. Charter's patient records were contained in the computer. Sanfiel testified that he reviewed this information and recalled that Charter was being investigated for defrauding the government. He contacted local law enforcement and the state attorney's office to initiate a criminal investigation. The agencies declined, telling him that the matter was outside their jurisdiction. Sanfiel then called the news media and allowed them to see the information concerning the patients. He asked that the patients' names be blurred to protect their identity. He told reporters that the hard drive contained the names of psychiatric patients, their admission dates, types of addiction, treatments, and psychiatric disorders. The story was broadcast along with the patients' names and diagnoses shown on the computer screen. One of the journalists located and interviewed a patient identified from Sanfiel's computer. The patient was distressed over the fact that his confidential medical information was being exposed to the public.

Sanfiel violated Florida Administrative Code by violating the confidentiality of information or knowledge concerning a patient. Florida Code Rule 59S-8.005 states in part that unprofessional conduct includes violating the confidentiality of information or knowledge concerning a patient. The board reasonably interpreted this provision to apply to the circumstances present in this case. Sanfiel knew that a nurse could be disciplined for disclosing such information, yet he intentionally released the information to the news media. It is reasonable to characterize Sanfiel's actions as unprofessional conduct.

Discussion

1. Describe why Charter patients had legal recourse for the unauthorized release of their medical information.
2. Describe what steps Charter could take to prevent similar occurrences in the future.

Requests by Patients

Patients have a legally enforceable interest in the information contained in their medical records and, therefore, have a right to access their records. Patients may have access to review and obtain copies of their records, x-rays, and laboratory and diagnostic tests. Access to information includes that maintained or possessed by a healthcare organization or a healthcare practitioner who has treated or is treating a patient. Organizations and physicians can withhold records if the information could reasonably be expected to cause substantial and identifiable harm to the patient (e.g., patients in psychiatric hospitals, institutions for the mentally disabled, or alcohol- and drug-treatment programs).

Failure to Release Patient Records

Failure to release a patient's record can lead to legal action. The patient, for example, in *Pierce v. Penman*[2] brought a lawsuit seeking damages for severe emotional distress when physicians repeatedly refused to turn over her medical records. The defendants had rendered different professional services to the plaintiff for approximately 11 years. The patient moved and found a new physician, Dr. Hochman. She signed a release authorizing Hochman to obtain her records from the defendant physicians. Hochman wrote a letter for her records but never received a response. The defendants claimed that they never received the request. The patient changed physicians again and continued in her efforts to obtain a copy of the records. Eventually, the defendants' offices were burglarized, and the plaintiff's records were allegedly taken. The detective in charge of investigating the burglary stated that he was never notified that any records were taken. The court of common pleas awarded the patient $2500 in compensatory damages and $10,000 in punitive damages. On appeal, the superior court upheld the award.

Requests by Third Parties

The medical record is a peculiar type of property because of the wide variety of third-party interests in the information contained in medical records. Healthcare organizations may not generally disclose information without patient consent. Policies regarding the release of information should be formulated to address the rights of third parties, such as insurance carriers processing claims, physicians, medical researchers, educators, and governmental agencies.

Privacy Exception

Criminal Investigation

The psychotherapist–patient privilege that exists under the federal rules of evidence can be overcome if the evidentiary need for a psychiatric history outweighs a privacy interest. In *In re Brink*,[3] the hospital sought to quash a grand jury request for the medical records pertaining to blood tests administered to a person under investigation. The court of common pleas held that physician–patient privilege did not extend to medical records subpoenaed pursuant to a grand jury investigation. A proceeding before a grand jury is considered secret in nature, inherently preserving the confidentiality of a patient's records.

Medicaid Fraud

Patient records may also be obtained during investigations into such alleged criminal actions as Medicaid fraud. The grand jury in *People v. Ekong*[4] was permitted to obtain certain patient files and records that were in the possession of the physician who was under investigation for Medicaid fraud. The physician contended that he could not release the files because of physician–patient privilege.

Substance Abuse Records

The federal Drug Abuse and Treatment Act of 1972[5] and the federal regulations promulgated thereunder provide that patient records relating to drug and alcohol abuse treatment must be held confidential and not disclosed except in specific circumstances. Unlike other medical records, drug and alcohol abuse records cannot be released until the court has determined whether a claimed need for the records outweighs the potential injury to the patient, to the patient–physician relationship, and to the treatment services being rendered. Because of these strict requirements, the courts have been reluctant to order the release of such records unless absolutely necessary.

Health Insurance Portability and Accountability Act (1996)

The Health Insurance Portability and Accountability Act (HIPAA) of 1996 (Public Law 104-191) was designed to protect the privacy, confidentiality, and security of patient information. HIPAA standards are applicable to all health information in all of its formats (e.g., electronic, paper, verbal). It applies to both electronically maintained and transmitted information. HIPAA privacy standards include restrictions on access to individually identifiable health information and the use and disclosure of that information, as well as requirements for administrative activities such as training, compliance, and enforcement of HIPAA mandates.

RETENTION OF RECORDS

The length of time medical records must be retained varies from state to state. For example, a California court revoked the license of a nursing facility for failure to keep adequate records. In *Yankee v. State Department of Health*,[6] the facility claimed that the word *adequate* was unclear and therefore the requirement was invalid. The court stated that the word *adequate* is not so uncertain as to render a penal statute invalid. Healthcare organizations, with the advice of an attorney, should determine how long records should be maintained, taking into account patient needs, statutory requirements, future need for such records, and the legal considerations of having the records available in the event of a lawsuit.

Retention of X-Rays: Failure to Preserve

The plaintiff in *Rodgers v. St. Mary's Hosp. of Decatur*[7] filed a complaint for damages against a hospital, alleging that the hospital breached its statutory duty to preserve for 5 years all of the x-rays taken of his wife. He alleged that the hospital's failure to preserve the x-ray was a breach of its duty arising from the state's x-ray retention act and from the hospital's internal regulations. The plaintiff asserted that because the hospital failed to preserve the x-ray, he was unable to prove his case in a lawsuit. The circuit court entered judgment in favor of the hospital, and the plaintiff appealed.

The Illinois Supreme Court held that a private cause of action existed under the x-ray retention act and that the plaintiff stated a claim under the act. The act provides that hospitals must retain x-rays and other such photographs or films as part of their regularly maintained records for a period of 5 years.

The hospital also argued that the loss of one x-ray out of a series of six should not be considered a violation of the statute. The court disagreed, finding that the statute requires that all x-rays be preserved, not just some of them.

COMPUTERIZED PATIENT RECORDS

Retaining all patient records for 5 years may seem unwieldy, but computers make the task feasible, while also increasing efficiency for many other information management processes. Healthcare organizations undergoing computerization must determine user needs, design an effective system, select appropriate hardware and software, develop user training programs, develop a disaster recovery plan (e.g., provide for emergency power systems and backup files), and provide for data security. Solid planning and design can lead to great achievements. Large medical centers are generating more than 100,000 orders a week. At the Brigham and Women's Hospital in Boston, laboratory and pharmacy results, pulmonary function, electroencephalography, and many other results-generating areas are based around the system. A strong aspect of the order-entry capability is its use of medical logic and medical expertise technology. The system flags cases where there have been duplicate physician orders and signals a patient allergy alert, resulting in an order cancellation.[8] Clearly, computers offer many advantages to today's health care.

Advantages

Computers have become an economic necessity and play an important role in assisting healthcare providers to improve the quality of health care. In the healthcare community, computers:

- Retrieve demographic information and consultants' reports, as well as laboratory, radiology, and other test results

- Improve productivity and quality

- Reduce costs

- Support clinical research

- Play an ever-increasing role in the education process

- Allow for interactive computer-assisted diagnosis and treatment

- Allow for computer-generated prescriptions (integrated computer systems and clinical pharmacy services are associated with reducing the incidence of medication errors)

- Generate reminders for follow-up testing

- Assist in the decision-making process

- Aid in standardizing treatment protocols

- Assist in the identification of drug–drug and food–drug interactions

- Are used in telecommunications around the world, transporting picture graphics (e.g., computed tomography scans) between nations

Disadvantages

Computers may be an economic necessity, but they are not perfect and have thus far proven to be costly investments. Computerization increases the risk of lost confidentiality and unauthorized disclosure of information. The rapid growth of the Internet has led to an explosion of high-technology crime and related illegal activities. Increases in cyber crime have led to a need for high-end technology products and services to combat these problems. Billions of dollars are spent annually to protect networks and critical infrastructures from cyber-based threats.

Legal Issues

Protecting a patient's medical information is an ongoing challenge; many federal laws protect credit information, but few protect the computerized medical record. In *Whalen v. Roe*,[9] the applicant, the commissioner of health of New York, had been enjoined by a three-judge court from enforcing certain provisions of the New York State Public Health Law that required the name and address of each patient receiving a schedule II controlled substance to be reported to the applicant. Schedule II drugs are those considered to have a high potential for abuse but also have an accepted medical use. Under the law, a physician prescribes schedule II drugs on a special serially numbered prescription form, one copy of which goes to the office of the New York commissioner of health where the data, including the name and address of the user, are transferred from the prescription form to a centralized computer file. The respondent claimed that mandatory disclosure of the name of a patient receiving schedule II drugs violated the patient's right of privacy and interfered with the physician's right to prescribe treatment for his or her patient solely on the basis of medical considerations. The court held that the patient identification requirement was the product of an orderly and rational legislative decision about the state's broad police powers. The statute does not impair any private interest on its face and does not impair the right of physicians to practice medicine free from unwarranted state interference.

MEDICAL RECORD BATTLEGROUND

The contents of a medical record must not be tampered with once an entry has been made; therefore, the record should be used wisely. Although the record should be complete and accurate, it should not be used as an instrument for registering complaints about another individual or the organization. Its purpose is to record the patient's course of care. Those individuals who choose to make derogatory remarks in a patient's record about others might find themselves in a courtroom trying to defend such notations in the record. Always consider that comments written during a time of anger may have been based on inaccurate information, which, in turn, could be damaging to one's credibility and future statements.

A nurse tends to access the medical record more often than other healthcare professionals, simply because of the greater amount of time spent with the patient. Because of the job description, the nurse monitors the patient's illness, response to medication, display of pain and discomfort, and general condition. The patient's care, as well as the nurse's observations, should be recorded on a regular basis. The nurse should comply promptly and accurately with the physician orders written in the record. A nurse who has doubt as to the appropriateness of a particular order should verify with the physician the intent of the prescribed order.

Licensure rules and regulations contained in state statutes generally describe the requirements and standards for the maintenance, handling, signing, filing, and retention of medical records. Failure to maintain a complete and accurate medical record reflecting the treatment rendered may affect the ability of an organization and/or physician to obtain third-party reimbursement (e.g., from Medicare, Medicaid, or private insurance carriers). Under federal and state laws, the medical record must reflect accurately the treatment for which the organization or physician seeks payment. Thus, the medical record is important to the organization for medical, legal, and financial reasons.

As noted in *Dodds v. Johnstone*,[10] during a physical exam conducted on October 30, 2000, the appellee indicated in her progress notes that she believed the appellant had been using cocaine prior to her last office visit. Appellee's notes read: "I believe by physical exam the patient was using cocaine on Friday before her office visit." The appellant filed a complaint in which she alleged that the appellee was negligent in her diagnosis of the appellant and that, as a result, she incurred a loss of compensation for her automobile accident claim and suffered severe emotional distress. The court reviewed the record of proceedings before the trial court and found that there was no genuine issue of material fact as to negligent infliction of severe emotional distress, loss of employment opportunities, or a decreased insurance settlement as a result of the notation in the patient's medical records.

FAILURE TO RECORD
PATIENT'S CONDITION

The plaintiff in *Gerner v. Long Island Jewish Hillside Med. Ctr.*[11] gave birth to her infant son at the defendant medical center. Dr. Geller, the attending pediatrician, arrived at the hospital 6 hours later. Geller, having noted and confirmed a slightly jaundiced condition, ordered phototherapy for the baby. After 3 days of treatment, the child's bilirubin count fell to a normal level, and Geller ordered the patient discharged. The child today is brain damaged, with permanent neurologic dysfunction.

The plaintiff alleged medical malpractice on the part of both the medical center and Geller for failing to diagnose and treat the jaundice in a timely manner. Following examination before trial, the medical center motioned and was granted summary judgment. The plaintiff and Geller appealed.

The New York Supreme Court, Appellate Division, held that questions of fact precluded summary judgment for the hospital. A number of allegations were raised as to negligence attributed solely to hospital staff. For example, notes of attending nurses at the nursery failed to record any jaundiced condition or any reference to color until the third day after birth, despite the parents' complaints to hospital personnel about the baby's yellowish complexion. Additionally, Geller ordered a complete blood count and bilirubin test as soon as he learned of the first recorded observation by a nurse of a jaundiced appearance. Test results, which showed a moderately elevated bilirubin count, were not reported by the laboratory until 10 hours after the blood sample was drawn, and another 3 hours passed before Geller's order for phototherapy was carried out. An issue was thus raised as to whether the 13-hour delay in commencement of the treatment was the proximate cause of the infant's injuries.

When handling medical records, professionals must recognize that intentional alteration, falsification, or destruction to avoid liability for medical negligence is generally sufficient to show actual malice. Punitive damages may be awarded whether or not the act of altering, falsifying, or destroying records directly causes compensable harm.

Falsifying Medical Records

The evidence in *Dimora v. Cleveland Clinic Foundation*[12] showed that the patient had fallen and broken five or six ribs; yet, upon examination, the physician noted in the progress notes that the patient was smiling and laughing pleasantly, exhibiting no pain upon deep palpation of the area. Other testimony indicated that she was in pain and crying. The discrepancy between the written progress notes and the testimony of the witnesses who observed the patient was sufficient to raise a question of fact. The court then considered the possible falsification of documents by the physician in an effort to hide the possible negligence of hospital personnel. The testimony of the witnesses, if believed, would have been sufficient to show that the physician falsified the record or intentionally reported the incident inaccurately in order to avoid liability for the negligent care of the patient.

The intentional alteration or destruction of medical records to avoid liability for medical negligence is sufficient to show actual malice, and punitive damages may be awarded regardless of whether the act of altering, falsifying, or destroying records directly causes compensable harm.[13]

Falsifying Business Records

Falsification of medical or business records is grounds for criminal indictment, as well as for civil liability. In *People v. Smithtown General Hospital*,[14] a motion to dismiss indictments against a physician and a nurse charged with falsifying business records in the first degree was denied. The surgeon was charged because he omitted to make a true entry in his operative report, and the nurse was charged because she failed to make a true entry in the operating room log.

Another such incident occurred in a rest home, where employees attempted to cover up the death of an elderly woman who had wandered away from the home and was found frozen in a drainage ditch.[15] The deceased patient had been brought back into the home, was dressed in a nightgown, and was placed in her bed. On the basis of the account given by employees, a physician signed the death certificate stating that the 77-year-old patient died in her sleep. An anonymous tip to the county examiner's office prompted an autopsy, and the patient was found to have frozen to death.

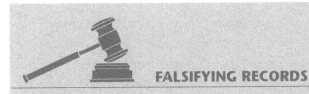

Citation: *Moskovitz v. Mount Sinai Med. Ctr.*, 635 N.E.2d 331 (Ohio 1994)

Facts

On November 10, 1987, Figgie removed a left Achilles tendon mass from Moskovitz. The tumor was found to be a rare form of cancer. A bone scan revealed that the cancer had metastasized.

Moskovitz's care was transferred to Figgie's partner, Makley, an orthopedic surgeon specializing in oncology at University Hospitals. Makley received Figgie's original office chart, which contained seven pages of notes documenting Moskovitz's course of treatment from 1985 through November 1987. Makley thereafter referred Moskovitz to radiation therapy at University Hospitals and sent along a copy of page 7 of Figgie's office notes to the radiation department at University Hospitals.

One month later, Makley's office forwarded the chart to Figgie's office; a copy was then sent to Moskovitz's psychologist. In January 1988, Makley's secretary requested that Figgie's office return the chart to Makley. At this time, it was discovered that the original chart had mysteriously vanished. The problem arose on October 21, 1988, when Moskovitz filed a complaint for discovery seeking to ascertain information relative to a potential claim for medical malpractice. Moskovitz claimed that she had never refused to have the tumor biopsied, but discrepancies in her medical record led to questions.

In his January 30, 1989, deposition, Makley produced a copy of page 7 of Figgie's office chart. That copy was identical to the copy ultimately recovered by the plaintiff's counsel from the radiation department records at University Hospitals. The copy produced by Makley contained a typewritten entry dated September 21, 1987, which stated: "Mrs. Moskovitz comes in today for her evaluation on the radiographs

reviewed with Dr. York. He was not impressed that [the mass on Moskovitz's left leg] was anything other than a benign problem, perhaps a fibroma. We [Figgie and York] will therefore elect to continue to observe."

However, Figgie's photostatic copy revealed that a line had been drawn through the sentence "We will therefore elect to continue to observe." The copy further revealed that beneath the entry, Figgie had interlineated a handwritten notation: "As she does not want excisional Bx [biopsy] we will observe." The September 21, 1987, entry was followed by a typewritten entry dated September 24, 1987, which states: "I [Figgie] reviewed the X-rays with Dr. York. I discussed the clinical findings with him. We [Figgie and York] felt this to be benign, most likely a fibroma. He [York] said that we could observe and I concur." At some point, Figgie also had added to the September 24, 1987, entry a handwritten notation, "see above," referring to the September 21, 1987, handwritten notation that Moskovitz did not want an excisional biopsy.

Figgie, at his deposition on March 2, 1989, produced records, including a copy of page 7 of his office chart. Because his original chart had been lost between December 1987 and January 1988, Figgie had made this copy from the copy of the chart that had been sent to Moskovitz's psychologist. The September 21, 1987, entry in the records produced by Figgie did not contain the statement "We will therefore elect to continue to observe." That sentence had been deleted (whited out) on the original office chart from which the psychiatrist's copy (and, in turn, Figgie's copy) had been made, in a way that left no indication on the copy that the sentence had been removed from the original records.

Figgie maintained that he did not discover the mass on the left Achilles tendon until February 23, 1987, and that Moskovitz continually refused a workup or biopsy.

During discovery, another copy of page 7 of Figgie's office chart, identical to the copy produced by Makley during his deposition, showed that the final sentence in the September 21, 1987, entry had been deleted from Figgie's original office chart sometime between November and mid-December 1987, the alteration presumably occurring while Figgie possessed the original chart.

Eventually, Figgie's entire office chart was reconstructed from copies obtained through discovery. The reconstructed chart contains no indication that a workup or biopsy was recommended by Figgie and refused by Moskovitz at any time prior to August 10, 1987.

In a videotaped deposition before her death, Moskovitz claimed that she never refused to have the tumor biopsied. The panel found in favor of the defendants participating in that proceeding with the exception of Figgie, and the trial court agreed. A panel of arbitrators unanimously found that:

3. The evidence supported a finding that plaintiffs' . . . decedent had a very good chance of long-term survival if the tumor was found to be malignant at a time when it was less than one centimeter in size. The evidence supported the fact that the tumor had not grown in size as of May 7, 1987. If Dr. Figgie had performed a biopsy prior to this date, the cancer would not have metastasized and the decedent would have recovered.

4. Dr. Figgie's office chart, which is the primary reference material in analyzing a physician's conduct, is filled with contradictions and inconsistencies.

5. Even if Dr. Figgie was first informed of the growth on February 23, 1987, he still fell below acceptable standards of care because he did not conduct further investigation until . . . X-rays performed in September 1987. All handwritten entries which appear on or prior to September 24, 1987, indicating that a biopsy was recommended or that the decedent refused further workup were subsequent changes of the records done

to justify Figgie's conduct. The sentence "We will therefore elect to continue to observe" on the September 21, 1987 entry was whited out and the handwritten entry "as she does not want excisional biopsy we will observe" was a subsequent alteration of the records. [*Id*. at 338]

The court of appeals upheld the finding of liability against Figgie on the wrongful death and survival claims. The court of appeals found that the appellant was not entitled to punitive damages as a matter of law. The court of appeals reversed the judgment of the trial court as to the award of damages and remanded the case for a new trial only on the issue of compensatory damages.

Issue

Is an intentional alteration or destruction of medical records to avoid liability sufficient to show actual malice? Can punitive damages be awarded regardless of whether the act of altering or destroying records directly causes compensable harm?

Holding

The Ohio Supreme Court held that the evidence regarding the physician's alteration of the patient's records supported an award of punitive damages, regardless of whether the alteration caused actual harm.

Reason

The intentional alteration or destruction of medical records to avoid liability for medical negligence is sufficient to show actual malice, and punitive damages may be awarded regardless of whether the act of altering, falsifying, or destroying records directly causes compensable harm. The jury's award of punitive damages was based on Figgie's alteration or destruction of medical records. The purpose of punitive damages is not to compensate a plaintiff, but to punish and deter certain conduct. The court warned others to refrain from similar conduct through an award of punitive damages.

Figgie's alteration of records exhibited a total disregard for the law and the rights of Moskovitz and her family. Had the copy of page 7 of Figgie's office chart not been recovered from the radiation department records at University Hospitals, the appellant would have been substantially less likely to succeed in this case. The copy of the chart and other records produced by Figgie would have tended to exculpate Figgie for his medical negligence while placing the blame for his failures on Moskovitz.

The intentional alteration or destruction of medical records to avoid liability for medical negligence is sufficient to show actual malice, and punitive damages may be awarded whether or not the act of altering, falsifying, or destroying records directly causes compensable harm.

Discussion

1. Discuss what procedure should be followed when clarifying an entry in a patient's medical record.
2. Is correction fluid helpful when clarifying medical record entries? Explain.

TAMPERING WITH RECORD ENTRIES

Closely related to falsification, tampering with records sends the wrong signal to jurors and can shatter one's credibility. Altered records can create a presumption of negligence.

Maintaining Integrity of Patient Records

The court in *Matter of Jascalevich*[16] held:

> We are persuaded that a physician's duty to a patient cannot but encompass his affirmative obligation to maintain the integrity, accuracy, truth and reliability of the patient's medical record. His obligation in this regard is no less compelling than his duties respecting diagnosis and treatment of the patient since the medical community must, of necessity, be able to rely on those records in the continuing and future care of that patient.

> Obviously, the rendering of that care is prejudiced by anything in those records, which is false, misleading or inaccurate. We hold, therefore, that a deliberate falsification by a physician of his patient's medical record, particularly when the reason therefore is to protect his own interests at the expense of his patient's, must be regarded as gross malpractice endangering the health or life of his patient.[17]

Dr. McCroskey faced a lawsuit for tampering with documents. The state board of medical examiners in a disciplinary hearing in *State Board of Medical Examiners v. McCroskey*[18] issued a letter of admonition to Dr. McCroskey based on a series of incidents arising out of the care of a patient's stab wound. Although the patient's condition was initially thought to be stable, he bled to death several hours after his admission to the hospital. McCroskey was the attending surgeon on the date of the incident and, therefore, responsible for the accurate completion of the patient's medical record. McCroskey declined to accept the letter of admonition, and a formal disciplinary hearing was held.

McCroskey erased and wrote over a preoperative note made by another physician concerning the patient's estimated blood loss. Specifically, the original record entry was completed by a surgical resident on the date of the patient's death and stated that the patient's blood loss just prior to surgery was "now greater than 3000 cc." Sometime after the autopsy, McCroskey changed the record to read that the patient's blood loss was "now greater than 2000 cc."[19] After listening to conflicting expert testimony, the administrative law judge (ALJ) concluded that the physician had not violated generally accepted standards of medical practice by adding the note to the patient's medical record days or weeks after the patient's death and then backdating the note to the date of the death.

On review of the ALJ's decision, the board accepted the ALJ's evidentiary finding that many physicians date a medical record entry to reflect the date of the medical event, rather than the date on which the entry was made. The board disagreed, however, with the ALJ's conclusion that this fact brought McCroskey's conduct within generally accepted standards of medical practice. Instead, the board determined that backdating a medical record entry falls below accepted standards of documentation. Having thus found two acts that fell below generally accepted standards of medical practice, the board concluded that McCroskey committed unprofessional conduct and issued a letter of admonition. On appeal, the court of appeals held that the board erroneously rejected the ALJ's findings. ·

On further appeal by the board, the Colorado Supreme Court held that the findings of the board were supported by substantial evidence. Because of the expertise of the board, it was in a position to determine the seriousness of the physician's conduct by placing the events in their proper factual context.

All three of the inquiry panel's witnesses testified that the generally accepted standard of practice requires that a medical record entry be dated with the date it is made. Even one of McCroskey's witnesses acknowledged that misdating the medical record was "certainly something that should not have been done." McCroskey did not simply backdate a trivial note in a patient's medical record. Instead McCroskey's actions took place in the context of a patient's death, which resulted in a coroner's autopsy, peer review activities, publicity, and several legal actions. McCroskey was the attending physician responsible for the accuracy of the patient's medical record, and yet he engaged in conduct that cast doubt upon the medical record's integrity. Under these circumstances, the Board was justified in considering McCroskey's conduct to violate the standard of care.[20]

Inaccurate Record Entries

Dimora,[21] a 79-year-old woman, was preparing to be discharged from the Cleveland Clinic. After using the toilet with the assistance of a student nurse, she lost her balance and fell backward. Dimora's broken ribs were not diagnosed until the following day, when x-rays were taken at Marymount Hospital.

A claim for punitive damages alleges that the clinic intentionally falsified Dimora's medical records or inaccurately and improperly reported the fall incident to avoid liability for its medical malpractice or negligence. The jury awarded a verdict in favor of Dimora in the amount of $25,000 for compensatory damages and $25,000 in punitive damages.

On appeal, the judgment of the trial court was affirmed. At trial, three witnesses testified that Dimora was crying and in pain approximately 45 minutes after the incident while she was still in the hospital. Testimony was offered that broken ribs would be painful upon deep palpation. The progress note of the examining physician at issue states in part:

Pt was in transport between walker and toilet seat according to student nurse. Pt was at walker and lost balance backward. The SN acted by holding the pt from the L side and gradually lowering her to the floor, and called for help. Pt was lifted back into wheelchair. On exam, pt has full use of all 4 extremities with good strength and no pain with movement. A small 5 × 8 cm area on the pts r posterior thorax was slightly scraped. It was

not tender to deep palpations and no crepitus was noted. There were no other lacerations, bumps or abrasions noted. Head was traumatic. The abrasion on the thorax was treated with lotion and ice. The pt was smiling and laughing pleasantly during the exam.

The discrepancy between the written progress notes and the testimony of the witnesses who observed Dimora was sufficient to raise a question of fact as to the possible falsification of documents by the physician to minimize the nature of the incident and the injury of the patient as a result of the possible negligence of clinic personnel. The testimony of the witnesses, if believed, would be sufficient to show that the physician falsified the record or intentionally reported the incident inaccurately to avoid liability for negligent care. If such evidence is believed, the jury could award punitive damages.

REWRITING AND REPLACING NOTES

Another temptation healthcare professionals should not fall prey to is the desire to clarify and explain one's activities in the care of a patient.

Nurse Changes Record Entries

In a well-publicized case that involved the death of a child, the nurse replaced her original notes with a second set of notes that were much more detailed and indicated that she had seen the patient more frequently than was reported in her original notes.[22] Rewriting one's notes in a patient's medical record casts doubt as to the accuracy of other entries in the record. It is easier to explain why one did not chart all activities than it is to explain why a new entry was recorded and an original note replaced.

ILLEGIBLE ENTRIES

Illegible handwriting is as ancient as the first stylus. Perhaps the simplest but one of the most potentially dangerous problems with medical records is illegible entries. Unfortunately, poor penmanship can cause injury to patients. The American Medical Association encourages physicians to print, type, or computerize physicians' orders. Medical errors because of poor handwriting can lead to extended length of hospital stays and, in some cases, the death of patients. A Harvard study found that "penmanship was among the causes of 220 prescription errors out of 30,000 cases."[23]

FAILURE TO MAINTAIN RECORDS

As with illegible penmanship, failure to maintain patient records may occur when a healthcare professional is busy, overwhelmed, or preoccupied. A disciplinary hearing was conducted in *Braick v. New York State Department of Health*[24] involving a physician by a hearing committee of the New York State Review Board for Professional Medical Conduct. The committee reviewed 122 specifications of misconduct, which included gross negligence, failure to adequately maintain patient records, and failure to obtain informed consent. The committee revoked the physician-petitioner's license. In reaching its decision, the committee found the bureau of professional medical conduct's expert credible, including his opinion that the physician was ultimately responsible for what happened to his patients during the relevant surgeries, and the committee rejected the efforts of the physician and his expert to shift responsibility to nurses.

The petitioner appealed to the administrative review board for professional medical conduct, which affirmed the committee's determination and penalty. On review by an appeals court, the physician's license was found to have been properly revoked.

IMPROPER RECORD KEEPING

Maintaining records, of course, does little good when the records are flawed with errors. In one such case, *Tulier-Pastewski v. State Board for Professional Medical Conduct*,[25] two hospital administrators testified and showed undisputed proof that the physician had recorded that a patient was alert during the purported examination when the patient was actually sedated and asleep. Evidence also indicated that the physician failed to properly document medical histories and current physical status. Although the physician asserted that evidence of failure to document did not support findings of negligence because there was no expert testimony that her omissions actually caused or created a risk of harm to a patient, an expert witness testified that the missing information as to certain patients was needed for proper assessment of the patient's condition and choice of treatment. This testimony, together with the obvious importance of cardiac information when treating patients with chest pain, provided a rational basis for the conclusion by administrative review board for professional medical conduct that the physician's deficient medical recordkeeping could have affected patient care. The physician was found to be practicing medicine negligently on more than one occasion. The record had supported the defendant's fraudulent practice.

CHARTING BY EXCEPTION

Some healthcare professionals institute a practice of charting by exception. On April 9, 1986, Borras, in *Lama v. Borras*,[26] while operating on Mr. Lama, discovered that the patient had an extruded disc and attempted to remove the extruded material. Either because Borras failed to remove the offending material or because he operated at the wrong level, the patient's original symptoms returned several days after the operation.

On May 15, Borras operated again but did not order preoperative or postoperative antibiotics. On May 17, a nurse's note indicated that the bandage covering the patient's surgical wound was extremely bloody, which, according to expert testimony, indicates the possibility of infection. On May 18, the patient was experiencing local pain at the site of the incision, another symptom consistent with an infection. On May 19, the bandage was soiled again. A more complete account of the patient's evolving condition was not available because the hospital instructed nurses to engage in charting by exception, a system whereby nurses did not record qualitative observations for each of the day's three shifts, but instead made such notes only when necessary to chronicle important changes in a patient's condition.

On May 21, Dr. Piazza, an attending physician, diagnosed the patient's problem as discitis—an infection of the space between discs—and responded by prescribing antibiotic treatment. Lama was hospitalized for several additional months while undergoing treatment for the infection.

After moving from Puerto Rico to Florida, Lama filed a tort action in the US District Court for the district of Puerto Rico. Although the plaintiff did not claim that the hospital was vicariously liable for any negligence on the part of Borras, he alleged that the hospital failed to prepare, use, and monitor proper medical records.

The jury returned a verdict awarding the plaintiff $600,000 in compensatory damages. The district court ruled that the evidence was legally sufficient to support the jury's findings, and an appeal was taken.

The US Court of Appeals for the First Circuit upheld the decision of negligence based on the charting-by-exception policy, but the jury had to decide whether the violation of the regulation was a proximate cause of harm to Lama.

Before deciding the case, the jury considered several important factors. For example, the jury may have inferred from evidence that, as part of the practice of charting by exception, the nurses did not regularly record certain information important to the diagnosis of an infection, such as the changing characteristics of the surgical wound and the patient's complaints of postoperative pain. Further, because there was evidence that the patient's hospital records contained described possible signs of infection that deserved further investigation (e.g., an excessively bloody bandage and local pain at the site of the wound), the jury could have reasonably inferred that the intermittent charting failed to provide the sort of continuous danger signals that would most likely spur early intervention by the physician.

CHARTING AND REIMBURSEMENT

When charting, professionals should be familiar with diagnosis-related groups (DRGs). DRGs refer to a methodology developed by professors at Yale University for classifying patients in categories according to age, diagnosis, and treatment resource requirements. It is the basis for the prospective payment system, contained in the 1983 Social Security Amendments for reimbursing inpatient hospital costs for Medicare beneficiaries. The key source of information for determining the course of treatment of each patient and the proper DRG assignment is the medical record. Reimbursement is based on preestablished average prices for each DRG. As a result of this reimbursement methodology, poor record keeping can precipitate financial disaster for a hospital. The potential financial savings for Medicare are substantial. Under this system of payment, if hospitals can provide quality patient care at a cost less than the price established for a DRG, they keep the excess dollars paid. This is an incentive for hospitals to keep costs under control. There is, however, a continuing fear that patients may, to their detriment, be discharged too early for financial reasons. This in turn leads to costly malpractice suits.

INCOMPLETE RECORDS: LOSS OF PRIVILEGES

Not only must the chart be accurate, but healthcare professionals must promptly complete records after patients are discharged. Persistent failure to conform to a medical staff rule requiring physicians to complete records promptly can be the basis for suspension of medical staff privileges, as was the case in *Board of Trustees Memorial Hospital v. Pratt.*[27]

LEGAL PROCEEDINGS AND THE MEDICAL RECORD

The ever-increasing frequency of personal injury suits mandates that healthcare organizations maintain complete, accurate, and timely medical records. The integrity and completeness of the medical record are important in reconstructing the events surrounding an alleged negligence in the care of a patient. Medical records aid police investigations, provide information for determining the cause of death, and

indicate the extent of injury in workers' compensation or personal injury proceedings.

When healthcare professionals are called as witnesses in a proceeding, they are permitted to refresh their recollections of the facts and circumstances of a particular case by referring to the medical record. Courts recognize that it is impossible for a medical witness to remember the details of every patient's treatment. The record therefore may be used as an aid in relating the facts of a patient's course of treatment.

If the medical record is admitted into evidence in legal proceedings, then the court must be assured the information is accurate, was recorded at the time the event took place, and was not recorded in anticipation of a specific legal proceeding. When a medical record is introduced into evidence, its custodian, usually the medical records administrator, must testify as to the manner in which the record was produced and the way in which it is protected from unauthorized handling and change.

The records purportedly relating to a patient's treatment in *Belber v. Lipson*[28] were not admissible as business records because the witness who had possession of them had no personal knowledge of the circumstances under which the records were prepared.

Whether such records and other documents are admitted or excluded is governed by the facts and circumstances of the particular case, as well as by the applicable rules of evidence. Admission of a business record requires "the testimony of the custodian or other qualified witness."[29] If a record can be shown to be inaccurate or incomplete or that it was made long after the event it purports to record, its credibility as evidence will be diminished.

CONFIDENTIAL COMMUNICATIONS

Beyond the medical record lies an even more complex issue within healthcare organizations: communication. The duty of an organization's employees and staff to maintain confidentiality encompasses both verbal and written communications and applies to consultants, contracted individuals, students, and volunteers. Information about a patient, regardless of the method in which it is acquired, is confidential and should not be disclosed without the patient's permission. All healthcare professionals who have access to medical records have a legal, ethical, and moral obligation to protect the confidentiality of the information in the records, as well as verbal communications between physicians and patients. Communication between individual physicians and communication that occurs in peer-review activities also fall under strict confidentiality procedures.

The Federal Health Care Quality Improvement Act of 1986[30] insulates certain medical peer-review activities affecting medical staff privileges from antitrust liability. Peer review is protected as long as there is reasonable belief that it is conducted in the furtherance of quality care. In enacting this legislation, Congress recognized that without such antitrust immunity, effective peer review may not be possible. Privileged communications statutes do not protect from discovery the records maintained in the ordinary course of doing business and rendering inpatient care. Such documents often can be subpoenaed after showing cause.

The burden to establish privilege is on the party seeking to shield information from discovery. The party asserting the privilege has the obligation to prove, by competent evidence, that the privilege applies to the information sought.

Breach of Physician–Patient Confidentiality

Patients enter the physician–patient relationship assuming that information acquired by physicians will not be disclosed, unless the patient consents or the law requires disclosure. Mutual trust and confidence are essential to the physician–patient relationship. An action alleging a breach of physician–patient confidentiality is analogous to invasion of privacy, and plaintiffs are entitled to recover damages, including emotional damages, for the harm caused by the physician's unauthorized disclosure.

In such a case, *Berger v. Sonneland,*[31] Berger revealed information during her initial appointment with Dr. Sonneland regarding her medical and personal history. When questioned about her personal history, Berger said that she had previously been married to Dr. Hoheim, a physician in Montana. She described her relationship with her ex-husband as extremely strained. After meeting with Berger, Sonneland contacted Hoheim and discussed Berger's use of pain medications. Based on information provided by Sonneland, Hoheim filed a motion in a Montana court seeking to modify the custody orders relating to the couple's two children.

Berger sought damages for Sonneland's breach of physician–patient confidentiality. The court granted Sonneland's motion for summary judgment based on the absence of damage evidence, concluding that Berger failed to establish any objective symptoms of emotional distress. Berger moved for reconsideration, urging the court to apply invasion of privacy principles rather than principles related to the tort of negligent infliction of emotional distress.

During the course of events in this case, an appellate court held that a tort action exists for damages resulting from the unauthorized disclosure of confidential information obtained within the physician–patient relationship. The court also held that there is sufficient evidence to raise a question of fact as to whether Berger was injured by Sonneland's unauthorized disclosure. The matter was remanded for further proceedings.

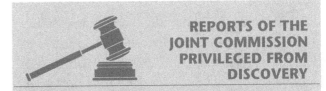

REPORTS OF THE JOINT COMMISSION PRIVILEGED FROM DISCOVERY

Citation: *Humana Hosp. Corp. v. Spears Petersen, 867 S.W.2d 858 (Tex. Ct. App. 1993)*

Issue

Are accreditation reports prepared by The Joint Commission privileged from discovery?

Facts

The plaintiff Garcia sued Dr. Garg for negligently performing an injection, battery, fraud, and lack of informed consent. Garcia also sued Humana Corporation for negligence in credentialing, supervising, and monitoring Garg's clinical privileges. The plaintiff's attorney requested documents from Humana, including reports prepared by The Joint Commission. The Joint Commission is a voluntary organization that surveys healthcare organizations for the purpose of accreditation.

Humana objected to releasing the reports of The Joint Commission and filed for a protective order preventing disclosure. The Joint Commission reports contained recommendations describing the hospital's noncompliance with certain of its published standards. Humana argued that The Joint Commission reports are privileged information under Texas statute. Under Texas law, the records and proceedings of a medical committee are considered confidential and are not subject to a court subpoena. The plaintiff argued that The Joint Commission is not a medical committee as defined in the Texas statute. The hospital's chief operating officer testified that the accreditation process with The Joint Commission is voluntary and the hospital chooses to have the accreditation survey. During the survey, The Joint Commission looks at certain quality care standards it has developed for hospitals. Humana argued that release of The Joint Commission's recommendations would do more than "chill" the effectiveness of such accreditation. The plaintiff argued that even if the information was privileged, it had already been disclosed to a third party, the hospital, thus waiving its rights to nondisclosure. The trial court denied Humana's motion for a protective order that, if granted, would have permitted it to withhold from discovery any information pertaining to credentialing, monitoring, or supervision practices of the hospital regarding its physicians. Humana appealed.

Holding

The Texas Court of Appeals held that the accreditation reports were privileged.

Reason

The purpose of privileged communications is to encourage open and thorough review of a hospital's medical staff and operations of a hospital with the objective of improving the delivery of patient care. The plaintiff argued that The Joint Commission is not a medical committee as defined in the Texas statute. The court of appeals found that the determinative factor is not whether the entity is known as a "committee" or a "commission" or by any other particular term, but whether it is organized for the purposes contemplated by the statute and case law. The Joint Commission is a committee made up of representatives of various medical organizations and thus fits within the statutory definition. It is organized for the purposes of improving patient care. Both Texas statute and case law recognize that the open, thorough, and uninhibited review that is required for such committees to achieve their purpose can only be realized if the deliberations of the committee remain confidential.

As to The Joint Commission's disclosing its report to the hospital, the only disclosure was to the hospital as the intended beneficiary of the committee's findings. The only disclosure made to the outside world was the accreditation certificate, which merely declares that the hospital has been awarded accreditation by The Joint Commission.

Discussion

1. Do you agree with the court's decision? Explain.
2. Discuss why privilege from discovery does not extend to all documents maintained in the normal course of business.

Privileged Information: Statements Protected

In *Estate of Hussain v. Gardner*,[32] discovery was sought regarding the statements given by a physician to the hospital's internal peer-review committee regarding the management and treatment of a patient. In this medical malpractice action, the plaintiff alleged that the defendant physician deviated from accepted medical standards in the care and treatment of the decedent during surgical procedures. The New Jersey Superior Court held that the statements given by the defendant were protected.

In a similar case, *Wylie v. Mills*,[33] the court adopted the privilege used in several federal jurisdictions that prevents disclosure of confidential, critical, evaluative, and deliberative material whenever the public interest in confidentiality outweighs an individual's need for full discovery. In applying the privilege to information contained in a corporate report on an accident in which an employee was involved, the court held that self-evaluation privilege protected the report from discovery. Without such protection, candid expressions of opinion or suggestions as to future policy would not be forthcoming as a result of a fear that these statements may be used against the employer in a subsequent litigation. The standard used for disclosure of confidential investigative records sets forth the following factors that should be taken into consideration: (1) the extent to which the information may be available from other sources; (2) the degree of harm that the litigant will suffer from its unavailability; and (3) the possible prejudice in the agency's investigation. The court adopted the holding that the plaintiffs had not made a strong showing of a particular need that outweighs the public interest in the confidentiality of the quality assessment committee. Because information is available from other sources, the court found that the information sought by the plaintiff was readily discoverable.

Credentialing Files Privileged

An action was filed against a healthcare provider in *Abels v. Ruf*[34] for the negligent credentialing of a physician who allegedly committed medical malpractice. The credentialing file relative to the physician in question was privileged. There was no dispute that the provider's credentialing documents fell within the scope of records of the provider's peer-review committee, and it was clear that the legislature had dictated that such documents were not obtainable from the provider. The Ohio Court of Appeals found that the trial court abused its discretion in ordering the appellant to provide certain credentialing documents to plaintiffs-appellees in discovery that may have been generated by the appellant's peer-review committee.

The trial court in *Hammonds v. Ruf*[35] erred when it ordered that certain portions of a physician's credentialing file be disclosed to medical malpractice plaintiffs because the documents were obtainable from original sources. The trial court abused its discretion in ordering the documents in question to be disclosed by the physician in violation of a clear statutory mandate prohibiting such disclosures.

Ordinary Business Documents

Privileged communications statutes do not protect from discovery the records maintained in the ordinary course of doing business and rendering inpatient care. Such documents often can be subpoenaed after showing cause.

Attorney–Client Privilege

Attorney–client privilege generally will preclude discovery of memorandums written to an organization's general counsel by the organization's risk management director. In *Mlynarski v. Rush Presbyterian–St. Luke's Medical Center*,[36] a memorandum written by the risk management coordinator to the hospital's general counsel was barred from discovery. There was undisputed evidence that the risk management coordinator had consulted with and assisted counsel in determining the legal action to pursue and the advisability of settling a claim that she had been assigned to investigate. Information contained in the memorandum was available from witnesses whose names and addresses were made available to the plaintiff. If the hospital later at trial decided to attempt to impeach those witnesses based on the coordinator's testimony, privilege would be waived and the hospital would be required to produce the relevant reports.

Committee Minutes Discoverable

When a plaintiff seeks case information that does not regard a committee's action or its exchange of honest self-critical study but, instead, regards merely factual accountings of otherwise discoverable facts, such information is not protected by any privilege because it does not come within the scope of information entitled to that privilege. This does not mean that the plaintiff is entitled to the entire study because it may contain evidence of policy making, remedial action, proposed courses of conduct, and self-critical analysis that the privilege seeks to protect in order to foster the ability of hospitals to regulate themselves unhindered by outside scrutiny and unconcerned about the possible liability ramifications that their discussions might bring about. As such, the trial court must make an in-camera inspection of such records and determine to what extent they may be discoverable.

In one such case, the plaintiff, a patient, brought an action against a hospital seeking to recover for injuries he sustained as a result of a nosocomial infection he allegedly contracted at the hospital.[37] The plaintiff claimed that his infection was a result of an act or omission on the part of the hospital in failing to protect him from such infections. During the discovery phase of the proceedings, the plaintiff filed a motion for production of documents seeking studies done by the hospital regarding the nosocomial infection rates per patients admitted. The hospital objected to this request, and the plaintiff obtained an order to compel the hospital to produce the documents. The court of appeal, on review, reversed the trial court's ruling, determining that statutes rendering hospital records confidential barred the information from disclosure.

The Louisiana Supreme Court, however, held that the records sought by the plaintiff were not entirely privileged from disclosure. The reliance of the court of appeal on La. R.S. 13:3715.3(A) and 44:7(D) was partially misplaced. These provisions were intended to provide confidentiality to the records and proceedings of hospital committees, not to insulate from discovery certain facts merely because they have come under the review of any particular committee. Such an interpretation could cause any fact that a hospital chooses to unilaterally characterize as privileged to be barred from discovery. The plaintiff sought facts relating to nosocomial infection rates in the defendant's hospital. A nosocomial infection is the same malady that gave rise to the plaintiff's injuries. Such facts would be highly relevant to the plaintiff's case or highly likely to lead to such evidence.

Peer-Review Documents Discoverable

The identity of peer-review committee members and individuals who may have given information to such committees is not always considered privileged. A state, for example, may access peer-review reports relating to a physician suspected of criminal negligence.[38] In a civil action, a hospital may be required to identify all persons who have knowledge of an underlying event that is the basis of a malpractice action, whether or not they were members of a peer-review committee.[39] The surgeon in *Robinson v. Magovern*[40] brought an action under the Sherman Antitrust Act, as well as under state law, seeking recovery because he had been denied hospital privileges. The plaintiff moved in the US District Court for an order compelling the defendants and certain third-party witnesses to respond to discovery requests and deposition questions. The defendants objected, claiming that the information sought was privileged and that the Pennsylvania Peer Review Protection Act seeks to foster candor and discussion at medical review committee meetings through grants of immunity and confidentiality. The court held that although there was a powerful interest in confidentiality embodied in the Pennsylvania Peer Review Protection Act, the act would not be applied to shield from discovery events surrounding the denial of staff privileges, including what occurred at meetings of the hospital's credentials committee and executive committee. The need for evidence was greater than the need for confidentiality in this case. The defendants' objections were overruled, and the motion to compel was granted.

In a similar case, the physician in *Ott v. St. Luke Hospital of Campbell County, Inc.*[41] brought a civil rights suit because his application for medical staff privileges was denied. The physician contended that he was not invited to several peer-review committee meetings or given an opportunity to be heard. The hospital filed for a protective order that would bar discovery of the proceedings of the peer-review committee. The hospital argued that such committees would become ineffective if their deliberations were discoverable and that the privilege claimed by the hospital is recognized in Section 311.377 of the Kentucky Revised Statutes Annotates (1990). The US district court held that where there was no real showing that the peer-review committee's functions would be impaired substantially, and where the benefit gained for correct disposal of the litigation by denying privilege was overwhelming, the hospital would not be permitted to assert privilege. The hospital's motion was therefore denied. The court indicated that it cannot permit the discharge of its responsibility to conduct a search for the truth to be thwarted by rules of privilege in the absence of strong countervailing public policies.

Staff Privileging Documents Discoverable

In *May v. Wood River Township Hospital*,[42] the patient's guardian sued the hospital and physicians, alleging that the hospital was negligent in providing care to the patient and in granting staff privileges to Dr. Marrese. The circuit court granted the guardian's motion and ordered the hospital to answer certain interrogatories. The hospital appealed.

The hospital submitted a memorandum of law and an affidavit stating that all documents concerning the granting of associate staff privileges to Marrese were kept for the purpose of improving the quality of patient care and were protected by the Illinois Code of Civil Procedure.

The trial court denied the hospital's motion for a protective order and granted the plaintiff's motion to compel, ordering the hospital to answer all of the plaintiff's interrogatories. The court determined that nothing related to work done, communications between executive committee members during their meetings, or discussions related to Marrese is protected; in addition, the minutes of the committee were also not protected as long as this information existed or was created before the actual decision to grant privileges to Marrese. The hospital urged on appeal, however, that no Illinois case has interpreted the code as being inapplicable to the credentialing process.

The Illinois Appellate Court held that the code of civil procedure did not protect information generated prior to the physician's application for staff privileges or his application for the privileges. The same is true of a host of materials that might be considered by the committee, for example:

- Whether staff privileges were granted, denied, or revoked at other hospitals

- Whether licenses to practice medicine were awarded, denied, suspended, or revoked in a given state

- Whether an applicant has ever been sued for malpractice

These facts would exist independent of a peer-review process. That which is nonprivileged cannot be converted to being privileged simply by handing the facts to a committee. On the other hand, if the committee sought to generate new opinions or information for consideration by the committee, a privilege could attach. For example, if the committee interviewed a colleague of Marrese's to elicit an opinion on Marrese's ability as a physician, that opinion could be privileged. If, however, the same opinion had been stated earlier in a deposition in a malpractice case and the committee reviewed the deposition, no privilege could attach to conceal the deposition from the discovery process.

Staff Credentialing Documents Not Discoverable

The underlying action in *McGee v. Bruce Hospital System*[43] involved a wrongful death claim. A circuit court order granted the plaintiffs a motion instructing the defendant, Bruce Hospital System, to produce the credentialing files and clinical privileges for each of the defendant physicians. The defendant physicians contended that such documentation is protected by South Carolina confidentiality statute [S.C. CODE ANN. § 40-71-20 (Supp. 1992)]. The trial judge found that the materials sought were discoverable.

On appeal, the South Carolina Supreme Court held that: (1) applications for staff privileges and supporting documents of appropriate training were protected by the confidentiality statute; (2) the confidentiality statute did not preclude discovery of general policies and procedures for staff monitoring; and (3) the patient could discover a listing of clinical privileges either granted or denied by the hospital. The overriding public policy of the confidentiality statute is to encourage healthcare professionals to monitor the competency and professional conduct of their peers in order to safeguard and improve the quality of patient care. The underlying purpose behind the confidentiality statute is not to facilitate the prosecution of civil actions but to promote complete candor and open discussion among participants in the peer-review process.

Section 40-71-20 of the South Carolina statute does not preclude the discovery of the general policies and procedures for staff monitoring. The information contained in the written rules, regulations, policies, and procedures for the medical staff would not compromise the statutory goal of candid evaluation of peers in the medical profession.

The outcome of the decision-making process is not protected. The confidentiality statute was intended to protect the review process, not to restrict the disclosure of the result of the process. Accordingly, the plaintiffs were entitled to a listing of clinical privileges either granted or denied by the hospital.

Search Warrant for Peer-Review Documents

In *In re Investigation of Liberman*,[44] long-term patient Liberman fell and injured her head while unattended. She later died, apparently as a result of complications from the fall. The attorney general (AG) commenced a criminal investigation into Liberman's death with more than 15 employees being questioned by the AG. The AG obtained and executed an investigatory search warrant for hospital documents. Before the documents left the hospital's premises, however, some of the documents were sealed because the hospital deemed them privileged peer-review documents.

A hearing was held in district court regarding the AG's motion for permission to unseal the documents. The district court was persuaded that the privilege statute asserted by the hospital did not apply because the documents were seized pursuant to a search warrant. The district court allowed the AG to unseal the documents, but the district judge stayed the decision to give the hospital an opportunity to appeal to the circuit court.

On appeal, the circuit court ruled that the peer-review documents were protected by peer-review privilege and that the privilege could be enforced even against documents seized pursuant to a search warrant. The court determined that the legislature intended the privilege to apply regardless of whether the documents were seized pursuant to a subpoena or a search warrant.

The Michigan statute MCL 333 § 21515 provides:

> (1) peer review information is confidential; (2) peer review information is to be used "only for the purposes provided in this article;" (3) peer review information is not to be a public record; and (4) peer review information is not subject to subpoena.

The legislation commands that a hospital maintain a peer-review process for the purpose of improving patient care. Allowing a prosecutor to obtain a hospital's peer-review materials pursuant to a search warrant would be to allow the prosecutor's general investigative powers to override the specific privilege of confidentiality that covers such materials. Accordingly, the Michigan Court of Appeals concluded that documents created by a peer-review body exclusively for peer-review purposes are not subject to disclosure pursuant to a search warrant in a criminal investigation.

HEALTH INSURANCE PORTABILITY AND ACCOUNTABILITY ACT

HIPAA was enacted by Congress in 1996. According to the Centers for Medicare and Medicaid Services, Title I of HIPAA protects health insurance coverage for workers and their families when they change or lose their jobs. Title II of HIPAA, the administrative simplification (AS) provisions, requires the establishment of national standards for electronic healthcare transactions and national identifiers for providers, health insurance plans, and employers. The AS provisions also address the security and privacy of health information. The standards are meant to improve the efficiency and effectiveness of the nation's healthcare system by encouraging the widespread use of electronic data interchange in health care.

Privacy Provisions

The HIPAA privacy provision took effect on April 14, 2003. Key privacy provisions include the following:

- Patients must be able to access their record and request correction of errors.

- Patients must be informed of how their personal information will be used.

- Patient information cannot be used for marketing purposes without the explicit consent of the involved patients.

- Patients can ask their health insurers and providers to take reasonable steps to ensure that their communications with the patient are confidential. For instance, a patient can ask to be called at his or her work number, instead of home or cell phone number.

- Patients can file formal privacy-related complaints to the US Department of Health and Human Services Office for Civil Rights.

- Health insurers or providers must document their privacy procedures, but they have discretion on what to include in their privacy procedure.

- Health insurers or providers must designate a privacy officer and train their employees.

- Providers may use patient information without patient consent for the purposes of providing treatment, obtaining payment for services, and performing the nontreatment operational tasks of the provider's business.

Security Provisions

The HIPAA security provisions took effect April 20, 2005. The security provision complements the privacy provision. HIPAA defines three segments of security safeguards for compliance: administrative, physical, and technical. Key provisions are as follows.

Administrative Safeguards

- Policies and procedures must be designed to clearly show how the entity will comply with the act.

- Entities that must comply with HIPAA requirements must adopt a written set of privacy procedures and designate a privacy officer to be responsible for developing and implementing all required policies and procedures.

- Policies and procedures must reference management oversight and organizational buy-in to comply with the documented security controls.

- Procedures should clearly identify employees or classes of employees who will have access to protected health information (PHI).

- Access to PHI in all forms must be restricted to only those employees who have a need for it to complete their job function.

- Procedures must address access authorization, establishment, modification, and termination.

- Entities must show that an appropriate ongoing training program regarding the handling of PHI is provided to employees performing health plan administrative functions.

- Covered entities that outsource some of their business processes to a third party must ensure that their vendors also have a framework in place to comply with HIPAA requirements.

- Care must be taken to determine if the vendor further outsources any data-handling functions to other vendors, while monitoring whether appropriate contracts and controls are in place.

- A contingency plan should be in place for responding to emergencies.

- Covered entities are responsible for backing up their data and having disaster recovery procedures in place.

- The recovery plan should document data priority and failure analysis, testing activities, and change control procedures.

- Internal audits play a key role in HIPAA compliance by reviewing operations with the goal of identifying potential security violations.

- Policies and procedures should specifically document the scope, frequency, and procedures of audits.

- Audits should be both routine and event based.

- Procedures should document instructions for addressing and responding to security breaches that are identified either during the audit or the normal course of operations.

Physical Safeguards

- Responsibility for security must be assigned to a specific person or department.

- Controls must govern the introduction and removal of hardware and software from the network.

- When equipment is retired, it must be disposed of properly to ensure that PHI is not compromised.

- Access to equipment containing health information should be carefully controlled and monitored.

- Access to hardware and software must be limited to properly authorized individuals.

- Required access controls consist of facility security plans, maintenance records, and visitor sign-in and escorts.

- Policies are required to address proper workstation use.

- Workstations should be removed from high-traffic areas, and monitor screens should not be in direct view of the public.

- If the covered entities use contractors or agents, they too must be fully trained on their physical access responsibilities.

Technical Safeguards

- Information systems housing PHI must be protected from intrusion.

- When information flows over open networks, some form of encryption must be used.

- If closed systems/networks are used, existing access controls are considered sufficient, and encryption is optional.

- Each covered entity is responsible for ensuring that the data within its systems have not been changed or erased in an unauthorized manner.

- Data corroboration, including the use of check sum, double-keying, message authentication, and digital signature, may be used to ensure data integrity.

- Covered entities must also authenticate entities with which it communicates.

- Authentication consists of corroborating that an entity is who it claims to be.

- Covered entities must make documentation of their HIPAA practices available to the government to determine compliance.

- Information technology documentation should also include a written record of all configuration settings on the components of the network because these components are complex, configurable, and always changing.

- Documented risk analysis and risk management programs are required.

CHARTING: SOME HELPFUL ADVICE

The medical record is the most important document in a malpractice action. Both the plaintiff and defendant use it as a basis for their actions and defense in a lawsuit. The following suggestions on documentation should prove helpful when charting in a patient's record.

- The medical record describes the care rendered to a patient. It should provide a clear timeline of patient care needs and how they were addressed from the time of admission to the time of discharge. It should include a complete and accurate medical history and physical, medications at the time of admission, allergies, over-the-counter drugs, vitamins, differential diagnoses, treatment plan, care rendered, and follow-up instructions.

- Medical record entries should be timely, legible, clear, and meaningful to a patient's course of treatment. Illegible medical records not only damage one's ability to defend oneself in a court action, but also can have an adverse effect on the credibility of other healthcare professionals who read the record and act on what they read.

- Progress notes should describe the symptom/s or condition/s being addressed, the treatment rendered, the patient's response, and status at the time inpatient care is discontinued. All notes must be dated and signed in order to provide an accurate history of the patient's care and treatment during the hospital stay. Follow-up on other caregiver notes should be described in the progress notes (e.g., observations of consultants, dietitians, nurses, pharmacists, physical therapists, and respiratory therapists).

- Long, defensive, or derogatory notes should not be written. Only the facts should be related. Criticism, complaints, emotional comments, and extraneous remarks have no place in the medical record. Such remarks can precipitate a malpractice suit.

- Erasures and correction fluid should not be used to cover up entries. Do not tamper with the chart in any form. A single line should be drawn through a mistaken entry, the correct information entered, and the correction signed and dated.

- Charts related to pending legal action should be placed in a separate file under lock and key. Legal counsel should be notified immediately of any potential lawsuit.

- A medical record has many authors. Entries made by others must not be ignored. Good patient care is a collaborative interdisciplinary team effort. Entries made by healthcare professionals provide valuable information in treating the patient.

- Reasoning for not following the advice of a consultant should be noted in the medical record, not so as to discredit the consultant, but to show the reasoning why a consultant's advice was not followed.

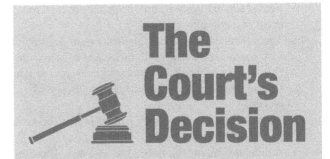

The Court's Decision

A West Texas jury ordered the physician, drugstore, and pharmacist to pay $225,000 to the family. The likelihood of similar occurrences is a growing danger as the number and variety of medications increase with similar names and look-alikes.

CHAPTER REVIEW

1. *Information management* is the process of facilitating the flow of information within and among departments and caregivers.
2. Healthcare organizations are required to maintain medical records for their patients in accordance with accepted professional standards and practices, and the requirements for these records are often set forth within each state's public health laws. Records should be complete, accurate, current, readily accessible, and organized.
3. An admission record contains data including age, address, reason for admission, Social Security number, marital status, religious affiliation, and other information required under federal and state requirements. It includes general consent and authorization for treatment forms. Patient-specific medical information is recorded in the clinical record.
4. Third-party reimbursement may be denied to an organization or physician who has failed to maintain a complete and accurate medical record. To receive federal funding, healthcare organizations must meet minimum federal standards for record keeping.
5. *Diagnosis-related groups* (DRGs) are a method of classifying patients by categories according to age, diagnosis, and treatment resource requirements. DRGs are the basis for the prospective payment system and are assigned using information detailed in a patient's medical record. Failure to keep complete and accurate records could result in difficulty in obtaining reimbursement.
6. Medical records are maintained for the benefit of the patients and are considered the property of the healthcare provider. Generally, healthcare professionals and healthcare organizations do not release medical records to patients. Most courts, however, take the view that patients have a right to access their records, and some states have issued legislation granting this access.
7. Records can be used as important evidentiary tools. The integrity and completeness of a medical record can be crucial in reconstructing the events surrounding alleged negligence.
8. The employees and staff of healthcare organizations are required to maintain the confidentiality of verbal and written communications. This is in accordance with both laws protecting a patient's right to privacy and ethical standards for healthcare professionals.
9. Lack of trust and confidence in a physician can destroy the integrity of the physician–patient relationship and negatively affect the quality and appropriateness of the treatment administered. Patients can be awarded damages if it is proven that a physician disclosed confidential information without authorization and that this disclosure resulted in harm to the patient.
10. The requirements for the length of time medical records must be retained differ among states. In determining the length of time records should be retained, organizations, along with advice from legal counsel, should consider patient needs, statutory requirements, future need for the records, and legal considerations of record availability in the event of a lawsuit.
11. The intentional alteration, falsification, or destruction of medical records to avoid liability for negligence is usually sufficient to show malice. Punitive damages may be awarded whether or not the act resulted in compensable harm. Falsification of medical or business records is grounds for both criminal indictment and civil liability.
12. Information can be shielded from discovery when the party that seeks to protect the information can establish privilege.
13. The restriction on disclosing patient information can be lifted under certain circumstances, including the information's relevance in a criminal investigation.
14. Although computers improve the ease and efficiency with which data are compiled and shared, they also pose confidentiality risks.
15. HIPAA requires the establishment of national standards for electronic healthcare transactions and national identifiers for providers, health insurance plans, and employers. HIPAA provisions also address the security and privacy of health information.

REVIEW QUESTIONS

1. What is information management as it relates to health care?
2. What are the basic purposes of the medical record?
3. Discuss the advantages and disadvantages of computer-generated medical records.
4. A medical record is the sole property of the patient and should never be released. Discuss your opinion on this statement.
5. What is the reasoning for the establishment of statutes that protect an organization's peer-review information?
6. Should statements given by a defendant to a hospital's internal peer-review committee be discoverable by a plaintiff? Explain your answer.
7. What records or parts thereof should be protected from discovery?
8. Should information gathered prior to a physician's application for staff privileges be privileged from discovery? Explain.
9. How long should patient records be maintained?

NOTES

1. Mimi Hall, "Doctor Held Liable for Fatal Handwriting Mix-Up," *USA Today*, October 21, 1999.
2. 515 A.2d 948 (Pa. Super. Ct. 1986).
3. 536 N.E.2d 1202 (Ohio Com. Pl. 1988).
4. 582 N.E.2d 233 (Ill. App. Ct. 1991).
5. 21 U.S.C. § 1175 (1972).
6. 328 P.2d 556 (Cal. Ct. App. 1958).
7. 597 N.E.2d 616 (Ill. 1992).
8. John P. Glaser, "Brigham and Women's Wager on Huge PC Network Pays Solid Returns," *Health Management Technology*, October 1994, at 7.
9. 423 U.S. 1313 (1975).
10. No. L-03-1303 (Ohio App. 2004).
11. 609 N.Y.S.2d 898 (N.Y. App. Div. 1994).
12. 683 N.E.2d 1175 (Ohio App. 1996).
13. *Moskovitz v. Mount Sinai Med. Ctr.*, 635 N.E.2d 331 (Ohio 1994).
14. 402 N.Y.S.2d 318 (N.Y. Sup. Ct. 1978).
15. "Deceit Found in Fatality at Rest Home," *New York Times*, February 5, 1995, at 35.
16. 442 A.2d 635 (N.J. Super. Ct. 1982).
17. *In re Jascalevich*, 182 N.J. Super. 445, 442 A.2d 635, 644–645 (1982).
18. 880 P.2d 1188 (Colo. 1994).
19. *Id.* at 1192.
20. *Id.* at 1196.
21. *Dimora v. Cleveland Clinic Foundation*, 683 N.E.2d 1175 (Ohio App. 1996).
22. Ronnie Greene, "Examiner: Treatment 'Appropriate,'" *The Miami Herald*, April 16, 1995, at 14A.
23. Esme M. Infante, "Doctors' Rx: Write Right," *USA Today*, June 14, 1994, at 1.
24. No. 94189 (N.Y. App. Div. 2004).
25. No. 94969 (Supreme Court of N.Y. App. Div. 2004).
26. 16 F.3d 473 (1st Cir. 1994).
27. 262 P.2d 682 (Wyo. 1953).
28. 905 F.2d 549 (1st Cir. 1990).
29. Federal Rules of Evidence, 28 § 803(6) (1988).
30. 42 U.S.C.A. § 11101–11152 (1989).
31. *Berger v. Sonneland*, 1 P.3d 1187 (2000).
32. 624 A.2d 99 (N.J. Super. Ct. App. Div. 1993).
33. 478 A.2d 1273 (N.J. Super. Ct. App. Div. 1984).
34. C. A. No. 22265 (Ohio App. 2005).
35. C. A. No. 22109 (Ohio Ct. App. 2004).
36. 572 N.E.2d 1025 (Ill. App. Ct. 1991).
37. *Smith v. Lincoln Gen. Hosp.*, 605 So. 2d 1347 (La. 1992).
38. *People v. Superior Court*, 286 Cal. Rptr. 478 (Cal. Ct. App. 1991).
39. *Moretti v. Lowe*, 592 A.2d 855 (R.I. 1991).
40. 521 F. Supp. 842 (W.D. Pa. 1981).
41. 522 F. Supp. 706 (E.D. Ky. 1981).
42. 629 N.E.2d 170 (Ill. App. Ct. 1994).
43. 439 S.E.2d 257 (S.C. 1993).
44. 646 N.W.2d 199 (Mich. App. 2002).

The Health Insurance Portability and Accountability Act (HIPAA): Not All About Health Insurance

Joan M. Kiel, PhD, CHPS, *Chairman University HIPAA Compliance and Associate Professor HMS, Duquesne University, Pittsburgh, Pennsylvania*

Chapter Objectives

- Develop an understanding of the circumstances leading to the passage of Health Insurance Portability and Accountability Act (HIPAA) and the several purposes that HIPAA is intended to serve.
- Examine the portions of HIPAA that are most pertinent to working managers, specifically the significant sections of the second of the five titles of HIPAA referred to in legislation as Administrative Simplification.
- Facilitate familiarization with the rules applicable in the implementation of HIPAA.
- Define the manager's role relative to the HIPAA Privacy Rule and Security Rules.
- Review the responsibilities incumbent upon the organization for the implementation of HIPAA and its maintenance as standard operating procedure.
- Review the potential uses of personal patient health information by the organization and define the circumstances governing the release of such information.

Introduction

The Health Insurance Portability and Accountability Act (HIPAA) is an important piece of federal legislation that has changed the way healthcare organizations do business. When it was initially being debated, healthcare managers feared the worst, thinking of added expenses. They surmised that they would have to add staff, and they thought that patients would be upset. Through it all, healthcare managers have had to make adjustments in operations and keep abreast of HIPAA. This chapter details HIPAA and describes how a healthcare manager can successfully implement the pertinent portions of this law.

History and Rationale

What patients tell physicians can sometimes consist of some of the most confidential information that pertains to themselves. They tell it to physicians with the understanding that it will be used for their medical care and will not be passed on to others who are not involved in their care. Unfortunately, this essential confidentiality is not always observed. Consider the following examples: Information discussed by a physician and a physical therapist in a less-than-private setting is overheard by visitors leaving the adjacent office of a social worker; written information is left on a computer screen in an open nursing station when a nurse answers a call light; or information is used for financial gain when facts about a well-known patient is sold to a tabloid publication. Additionally, information stored electronically has the potential to be sent to many people with the click of a computer stroke, necessitating the implementation of security systems to prevent "healthcare hacking." Whether perpetrated purposefully or inadvertently, scenarios such as those discussed has led to federal legislation to protect patient health information.

HIPAA was enacted in part to protect the privacy, security, and confidentiality of patient health information. It also ensures secure transactions and assigns identifiers for providers, insurers, and patients to ease administrative transactions. HIPAA exists for both for the patient and the healthcare delivery system so that confidential information is utilized as it should be for the care of the patient and so that administrative transactions can be completed effectively and efficiently.

HIPAA, or Public Law 104-191, contains five titles addressing various areas of responsibility:

1. Healthcare Access, Portability, and Renewability
2. A. Preventing Healthcare Fraud and Abuse
   B. Medical Liability Reform
   C. Administrative Simplification
3. Tax-Related Health Provision
4. Group Health Plan Requirements
5. Revenue Offsets

Contained within the Administrative Simplification section of Title II are the three main areas that are pertinent to most healthcare managers: electronic data interchange, which includes transactions, identifiers, and code sets; privacy; and security. To further delineate these three main areas, HIPAA is divided into 11 rules. It is from these rules that healthcare managers then develop policies and procedures to ensure compliance with the law.

The 11 Rules of HIPAA

The first portion of HIPAA, Transactions and Code Sets, was scheduled for compliance by October 16, 2002. As of October 16, 2009, just 6 of the 11 rules of HIPAA had been released for implementation with compliance dates. Thus, for healthcare managers, HIPAA implementation will be an ongoing process for some time to come. The 11 rules are as follows:

1. The **Claims Attachment Standards Rule** establishes national standards for the format and content of electronic claims attachment transactions (proposed in the September 23, 2005 Federal Register).

2. The **Clinical Data Rules/Electronic Signature Standard** establishes national standards for clinical data and data transmission.

3. The **Data Security Rule** establishes physical, technical, and administrative protocols for the security and integrity of electronic health data (April 20, 2005).

4. The **Enforcement Rule** establishes rules for how the government intends to enforce HIPAA (February 15, 2006).

5. The **Standard Transaction for First Report of Injury Rule** establishes national standards for the format and content of electronic first-report-of-injury transactions used in Workers' Compensation cases.

6. The **Standard Unique Identifier for Employers Rule** establishes the federal tax identification number as an employer's national unique identifier (July 30, 2004).

7. The **Unique Identifier for Individuals Rule** mandates a single patient identifier for all of an individual's patient health information.

8. The **Standard Unique National Health Plan/Payer Identifier Rule** establishes a national identifier for each health insurer.

9. The **Standard Unique Healthcare Provider Identifier Rule** establishes a national identifier for each provider (May 23, 2007).

10. The **Privacy Rule** establishes guidelines for the use and disclosure of patient health information (April 14, 2003).

11. The **Transactions and Code Sets Rule** establishes standard formats and coding of electronic claims and related transactions (October 16, 2002 or 2003).[1]

A Manager's Guide to the HIPAA Rules

As healthcare managers had just passed beyond the Y2K flurry of activity, the first rule of HIPAA, Transactions and Code Sets, was being released for implementation. The required implementation date was October 16, 2002, although covered entities were able to request a 1-year extension. As part of HIPAA's mission to ease electronic transactions, this rule focused on the development of standardized formats for electronic claims and their related transactions. HIPAA also specified what a HIPAA transaction was.

1. Healthcare claims or equivalent transactions
2. Healthcare payment and remittance advice
3. Coordination of benefits
4. Healthcare claim status
5. Enrollment and disenrollment in a health plan
6. Eligibility for a health plan
7. Health plan premium payments
8. Referral certification and authorization
9. First report of injury
10. Health claims attachments
11. Other transactions that the secretary may prescribe by regulation[2]

Healthcare managers need to be aware that as the revised *International Classification of Diseases (ICD-10)* is introduced (projected for Fall 2011), these transactions may undergo some changes. But all have the common objective of facilitating more accurate and efficient transactions.

The next rule to be implemented came with much fanfare (as opposed to the Transactions and Code Sets, which arrived quietly), as it impacted patients directly. With Transactions and Code Sets, patients do not know how their medical diagnoses are being coded, nor is it a great concern to them (as long as the bill is paid by the insurer). With the Privacy Rule, however, patients have forms to sign and new policies to adhere to with regard to accessing their health information.

The covered entity must employ an individual designated as a privacy officer. This person can be full time or part time, but must be intimately knowledgeable of HIPAA. It is certainly not a position to be given to someone in title only. This person is responsible for understanding and implementing the Privacy Rule. Although no specific background is required of the privacy officer, the person must have an understanding of health information, information technology, regulatory compliance, and management.

The first big change for both the staff and the patients was the introduction of the Notice of Health Information Privacy Practice, simply called the Notice. Employees of the covered entity have been required to provide the Notice once to every patient seen on or after April 14, 2003. On February 17, 2009, the Health Information

Technology for Economic and Clinical Health Act (HITECH) made changes to the Notice; thus on and after February 17, 2010, the revised Notice must be provided to all patients once. This is to be remembered concerning the HIPAA Privacy Rule: Whenever the Notice is revised by any legislation, it must again be provided to all patients.[3] It is necessary to have a process in place, whether paper or electronic, to keep track of who has been given the Notice and who has not. For example, if a long-standing patient does not present at the office again until 2012, the system must indicate that this patient has not been in since before February 17, 2010 and thus must receive the revised Notice. On the other hand, one should not wish to waste time and money or irritate the patients by repeatedly giving them the Notice. The Notice must also be changed on the provider's website and in any postings within the facility. Managers must also budget for the costs of keeping the Notice current.

Patients will also see new forms when they request copies of their medical information. The Privacy Rule has altered the standard Release of Information Form, although it remains unchanged in its essential contents. Patients also have the opportunity to request to amend their medical records, and forms must be completed for this purpose. Once completed, forms are reviewed by the author of the medical record notes or perhaps others if the original writer is not available. The privacy officer must be able to lead this process and ensure that all HIPAA documents are retained for 6 years. This in itself takes planning as one must decide whether records will be stored on-site or off-site, and electronically or on paper. A sample request form is shown in Exhibit 1.

Not all information is to be retained. Material that is not to be kept must be disposed of in a manner that ensures it cannot reasonably be reproduced. For paper, the most popular disposal method is shredding. For electronic data, the most popular way is degaussing. For either method, however, the covered entity must have a policy in place. If an external firm is used for disposal, it must provide the covered entity with certificates of destruction stating that they did in fact destroy the data and did not retain it or pass it on to others. A certificate of external destruction is shown in Exhibit 2.

A significant requirement that encompasses the entire covered entity involves the knowledge and awareness of HIPAA by all workforce members. All must be trained about HIPAA, and that training must be documented. In addition to training, HIPAA awareness must be routinely reinforced. This provision was put in place so that HIPAA is not forgotten, but rather remains a part of standard operating procedures. At every staff meeting the healthcare manager can simply have HIPAA on the agenda and review its status and implementation. The manager can review with the privacy officer how processes and procedures are being carried out and what their apparent effects are on the entity.

Employees must also be aware of their limits on access to information. Based on one's role, employees will be allowed to have access to only the information they need to fulfill their roles and nothing more. The need to know and minimum necessary standards apply such that employees do not acquire patient health information over and above what is needed to complete the task at hand.

Exhibit 1

Request for Amendment of Health Information

Patient name: _____

Medical record number: _____

Birth date: _____

Address: _____

Date of information to be amended: _____

Type of information to be amended: _____

Why is the information inaccurate or incomplete? _____
_____
_____

What should the information say? _____
_____
_____

If the request is agreed upon, where else should the amended information go?

Name: _____

Address: _____

_____   _____
Signature of patient   Date

To Be Completed by the Healthcare Provider:

Date received: _____

By whom: _____

Request for amendment has been: ACCEPTED   DENIED

If denied, state reason: _____
_____

Information is accurate and complete

Healthcare provider's reason: _____
_____
_____
_____
_____

_____   _____
Signature of healthcare provider   Date

Exhibit 2

Destruction of Patient Health Information by an External Entity

Name of facility and address: _____

Vendor name and address: _____

Description of information, and time period of the information: _____

Pick-up date of material: _____

Quantity of information destroyed: _____

Date of destruction: _____

Method of destruction: _____

Name of person doing destruction: _____

Signature: _____   Date: _____

As stated in the Notice of Health Information Privacy Practices, a patient has the right to file a HIPAA compliant with the covered entity, usually directly with the privacy officer. The first duty of the privacy officer—and this is where that official really needs to know HIPAA thoroughly—is to determine whether the complaint is truly HIPAA related. The patient cannot use the HIPAA complaint process, for example, to complain about waiting too long to see a physician. The covered entity must have a complaint process in place directing where and how patients can file complaints to how these are to be investigated and processed. If a complaint is warranted, sanctions must be assessed against the involved employees.

Not only do complaints warrant follow-up, but routine HIPAA audits may also reveal something that is not HIPAA compliant. Although the HIPAA Privacy Rule does not specify how often audits are to be performed, the healthcare manager can base HIPAA audit frequency on the timing of other audits such as those for billing and quality assurance. Areas in which issues arise are of course audited more frequently. It is necessary to document the audits and their findings; any adverse findings must be addressed via a documented action plan with subsequent follow-up on results.

Healthcare managers need to work with their privacy officer in relation to two external groups: business associates and researchers. Business associates are external constituents who see the covered entities personal health information but are not part of the organization's workforce (e.g., a computer vendor or an outside billing company). With such associates there must be a signed business-associate agreement calling for compliance with all HIPAA regulations. Under HITECH, implemented February 17, 2010, business associates must adhere to all of the HIPAA Security policies and not simply provide reasonable assurance that they are keeping patient health information private, secure, and confidential. The covered entity must also remain in communication with business associates to ensure that any noncompliance is corrected immediately and is not as a result of malice.

Persons conducting research in your organization and using personal health information also must be compliant with HIPAA. Data used for research cannot compromise the privacy, security, and confidentiality of patient health information.

The healthcare manager, in concert with the HIPAA privacy officer, must be proactive in protecting patient health information. Whether involving house staff, patients, themselves, business associates, or researchers, there is always much to be attended to and monitored under the HIPAA Privacy Rule.

Following the Privacy Rule is the HIPAA Security Rule, implemented April 20, 2005. The Security Rule is unique in including both required and addressable policies, thus it is entity dependent. Covered entities must follow the implementation specifications for the required policies. With the addressable policies, a covered entity must assess whether each implementation specification is reasonable and appropriate for protecting its patient health information.[3] The policies are then further divided into the three categories of technical, administrative, and physical aspects of security.

Just as the Privacy Rule calls for a privacy officer, a security officer is required for the Security Rule. This can be the same person as the privacy officer, as long as the individual has the time and expertise to cover both roles. Employees must be trained in security measures and this training must be documented. Security awareness among employees must also be stressed throughout the organization.

Documentation is vital concerning the Security Rule. Just as with privacy documentation, all HIPAA security documentation must be retained for 6 years. The Security Rule also necessitates a disaster manual documenting procedures to follow in the event of a disaster during which health information could be in jeopardy. This manual should exist in concert with the emergency-mode-operation plan intended to keep the organization functioning to the best of its ability in any compromised situation. The security officer, often the primary author of the manual, must be thoroughly conversant with its contents at all times. The security officer will most likely also be the person who implements the security incident policy. Table 1 lists the necessary security policies.

Table 1 *Areas of Necessary Security Policy Coverage*

Security Policies	Administrative	Physical	Technical
Required	1. Risk Analysis/Assessment 2. Risk Management 3. Sanction Policy/Disciplinary System 4. IS Activity Review 5. Assigned Security Responsibility (Security Officer) 6. Workforce/Personnel Security 7. Clearinghouse Functions/ Hybrid Entity 8. Response and Reporting 9. Data Backup Plan 10. Security Plan 11. Critical Business Processes/ Contingency Plan 12. Business Associates 13. Evaluation	1. Workstation Security 2. Device and Media Controls 3. Disposal of Computers 4. Media Reuse	1. Unique User Identification 2. Emergency Access 3. Audit Trails 4. Person or Entity Authentication
Addressable	1. Authorization and/or Supervision of Access to personal health information Personal Health Information (PHI) 2. Access to Data/Workforce Clearance 3. Terminating Access 4. Granting Access/Access Control 5. Access Establishment and Modification/Personnel Security 6. Security Reminders/Awareness 7. Malicious Software 8. Log-in Monitoring 9. Password Management 10. Testing and Revision 11. Applications and Data Criticality	1. Disaster Recovery/ Restore Lost Data 2. Physical Safeguards 3. Access Control & Validation 4. Maintenance Records/Logs 5. Accountability/ Transfer of Media & 6. Copy electronic personal health information.	1. Automatic Log Off 2. Encryption and Decryption Mechanism 3. Authentication of Electronic PHI 4. Integrity Controls 5. Encryption of Transmitted PHI

The security officer must be the person who implements and monitors policy compliance. The HIPAA Rule does not prescribe specific security measures, but rather provides blanket mandates and allows the organization to decide how these will be met. For example, the organization must have authentication methods in place, but whether these include passwords, thumbprints, or retinal scans is the organization's decision.[3]

Since access to patient health information is role-based, access-control audits must be completed. Employees who do not need access to information to perform their jobs will be identified on an audit if they violate access rights. With electronic records violations are readily detectable as one can look at the computer history, but with paper records there is more reliance on one's word that another was seen with the record. Computers should clearly record that electronic records are audited when one logs in. The computer should also have an automatic log-off process in the event of an emergency. Employees should never share their passwords except in a true emergency, nor should they store their passwords in obvious places.

When an employee leaves the organization either voluntarily or involuntarily, access must be terminated. It is particularly important when an employee is terminated involuntarily, as time is of the essence to prevent the terminated employee from saving any files for personal use or destroying files. If at all possible, a terminated employee's computer should be examined for any such activity before the person's departure. Thus another function of the security officer or designee is to have all files backed up as a precaution against loss.

In the same manner as the privacy officer, the security officer needs to manage the business-associate agreements. The same method used with the Privacy Rule can be used here.

Although the Security Rule is fairly extensive, its presence it is not nearly as evident to the patient as is the Privacy Rule.

The final three rules, the Standard Unique Employer Identifier Rule, the National Provider Identifier Rule, and the Enforcement Rule are not as extensive as the Privacy and Security Rules but they are just as important from a managerial perspective. The Standard Unique Employer Identifier Rule was implemented July 30, 2004. This rule calls for the organization to use its employer identification number (EIN) as its standard identifier. Many organizations were already doing this before HIPAA, so compliance was not an issue. For those who were not doing so, it was a matter of replacing what they had been previously using with the EIN.

The National Provider Identifier Rule was implemented May 23, 2007. This rule required healthcare providers to use a 10-digit unique identifier. The covered entities had to apply for the numbers and ensure they were used in all transactions. Computer fields, as well as forms, and policies needed to be updated. Inventorying the locations where the numbers are used is itself a large task.

The Enforcement Rule was implemented on February 16, 2006. As its name indicates, this rule mandates enforcement of HIPAA. Healthcare managers had to develop appropriate policies and procedures. This rule specifies what happens if there is a violation of HIPAA; it describes the issues of evidence and trial situations. Mangers need to understand this rule in the unlikely event of ever being a defendant or a plaintiff or involved in some other way in a legal debate.

These six rules of HIPAA currently set the stage for the remaining five rules. The healthcare manager will utilize the same skills and processes in implementing the remaining five as applied in the implementation of the first six. Most importantly, managers must come to view HIPAA as a part of standard operating procedures.

What Organizations Need to Do for All Six Implemented Parts

With 6 of the 11 rules of HIPAA released and 5 more to go, healthcare managers need to see HIPAA as an essential part of general operations. If its inevitability is recognized and it is incorporated into how one regularly does business, it will not feel like a legal albatross. Its integration into standard operating procedure requires putting some specific things in place.

First, as stated for the Privacy and Security Rules, a covered entity must employ a privacy officer and a security officer. Once in place, this person or persons can then, in concert with the healthcare manager, implement and manage HIPAA. A sample job description for a privacy officer appears in Exhibit 3.

The privacy and security officer is supported by a HIPAA committee. The HIPAA committee is comprised of people from information technology, health information management, administration, human resources, finance, and research if applicable. All of the parts of HIPAA must be represented on the HIPAA committee and thus a wide variety is needed in the committee's membership.

The third and most time-consuming responsibility is the development of the policies and procedures needed for all of the HIPAA rules. These policies are best developed from the law itself rather than from secondary sources. In this manner, the organization will be using the most precise policy language. Also, as with the Security Rule's addressable policies, all organizations will not be the same in size and scope so it is preferable to avoid using policies from other organizations. Each HIPAA rule should be covered by a policy manual or at least a separate manual section for easy reference. In drafting one's own, the organization will also be able to include consideration of implementation and changes to business operations. The HIPAA committee can be most helpful in drafting polices. In addition, many organizations have a policy committee that can also assist.

The fourth responsibility requires the covered entity to provide a training and awareness program for all workforce members. Not only as each part of HIPAA is unveiled must there be training, but this training must also be ingrained into the fabric of the organization. It cannot be a do-it-once and forget-about-it event. Training can be done in-house or outsourced; it can be done face-to-face, via computer, or by distance education. In the majority of small- to medium-sized organizations, it is the role of the privacy and security officers to perform this task. In larger organizations, online training is used or is outsourced to trainers so that it will not take up all of the time

Exhibit   3

Sample Job Description, Privacy Officer

Title: Privacy Officer
Division: Corporate Administration
Reports to: Chief Executive Officer of the covered entity
Position purpose: The privacy officer is responsible and accountable for all activities related to the development, implementation, evaluation, and modification of activities concerning the privacy of and access to patient health information as designated by HIPAA.

Position responsibilities:

- Identify, implement, and maintain organizational patient health information privacy policies and procedures.
- Work with the security officer, compliance committee, management, and staff in ensuring that privacy and security policies and procedures are maintained.
- Is responsible and accountable for all activities related to the privacy of and access to patient health information.
- Perform health information privacy risk assessments.
- Perform ongoing compliance monitoring activities and works with management to operationalize these monitoring activities into the daily functions.
- Develop and implement compliance related forms.
- Develop and maintain initial and ongoing training for all workforce members of the organization on HIPAA and HITECH.
- Review and bring into compliance all business associate agreements in regards to HIPAA and HITECH.
- Establish and implement a system to track assess to patient health information.
- Establish and implement a process allowing patients the right to inspect and request to amend their health information.
- Establish a program whereby complaints can be received, documented, tracked, and investigated.
- Develop a disciplinary system of sanctions for failure to comply with HIPAA for employees and constituents of the organization.
- Promote an ongoing culture of information privacy awareness and compliance to all related policies and laws.
- Develop policies and procedures for release of information and access to information.

- Maintain current knowledge of applicable federal, state, local, and organizational privacy laws and regulations.
- Work with all facilities and departments to standardize policies and procedures in regards to the privacy of patient health information.
- Lead the compliance committee and amend it as needed.
- Communicate as often as necessary due to changing regulations and compliance issues.
- Perform other activities as assigned.

Position qualifications:
- Bachelor's degree in a healthcare-related field is required.
- Certification in Healthcare Privacy and Security is recommended.
- Three years of management experience in health care.
- Knowledge of information privacy laws and issues related to access to health information, release of information, and patient rights.

of the privacy and security officers. All of the training must be documented and the documentation must be retained for 6 years. Some more thoughtful managers simply put it in the employee files and keep it beyond 6 years as long as the person remains employed. Training is done as changes occur to HIPAA, but sustained awareness must to be a regular business practice. Simply having a discussion at a staff meeting on HIPAA may constitute awareness; therefore, this activity need not be extensive to be effective. Of course if there is a violation, training must address that in the correction plan. Training is never ending, as HIPAA itself must be regarded as never ending.

The fifth responsibility concerns the development of a document retention system to retain all HIPAA materials for a minimum of 6 years. At the onset, many thought that this would be easy: Simply save everything. But doing so eventually becomes overwhelming in the face of the need to retrieve a specific record, thus the need for an organized method of retention.

HIPAA materials that must be retained include the forms that patients, employees, and business associates complete, policies that are revised, employee records such as for training and sanctions, audits and updates, and any material that contains patient health information that may not exist in the formal medical record (e.g., research forms). As a first step, a documentation retention subcommittee of the HIPAA committee can be formed. It is this group's responsibility to determine what needs to be retained and who has it, and then determine the quantity of information to save and whether its form be paper, electronic, or audio. Multiply that effort by 6 years and then determine how and where the material can be saved. For example, can paper be scanned? Or will the paper be saved in hard copy but perhaps off-site? Here budgetary considerations emerge. Initially many managers did not consider processing and retention costs; the amount of material that must be saved can be large. Also, if one contracts with an off-site storage organization, it is necessary to reckon with the cost of retrieval. How much per piece? How much per retrieval trip? Retention is not simply saving items; it necessarily includes an understanding of the process of doing business.

The sixth responsibility concerns development and implementation of an audit system. This was much more prominent when the Enforcement Rule was implemented. The basic assumption is that if it is not documented, it was not done. Unfortunately, one's word is never good enough when the healthcare manager must respond to a HIPAA complaint. Making audits a part of standard operating procedures shows that the organization is serious about it, and that, in itself, helps create a culture of caring and competency. A sample audit report form is shown in Exhibit 4.

Exhibit 4

Sample Audit Report Form

Date of audit: _____

Audit performed by: _____

Subject of audit: **Please circle subject of audit**
Computer log-ins
Medical record documentation
Coding and billing (claim denials)
Adherence to confidentiality policies
Adherence to security policies
Update of employee files
HIPAA training of employees
Review of violations/operational issues
Review of personnel access to patient health information
Number of breach of confidentiality issues
Claim denials
Other: _____

Department audit took place in: _____

Sample of employees surveyed: Number: _____ Type: _____

Adherence percentage: _____

Nonadherence percentage: _____

Report rationale: _____

Action plan:
_____
_____

The next responsibility calls for development and posting of a complaint process. Any patient has the right to file a HIPAA complaint if he or she believes that something that occurred is not consistent with HIPAA requirements. This must be clearly stated in the notice, which must also delineate the process for filing a complaint both internally and with the federal government. The healthcare manager must take every complaint seriously and ensure it is investigated. The manager, along with the HIPAA privacy officer, must first determine if a complaint is actually HIPAA related. If so, the privacy officer will further investigate and also call in the security officer if the complaint involves security issues. If not HIPAA related, the complaint goes back to the manager for follow-up as a general personnel issue. Complaints must be tracked such that employee follow-up occurs, it is determined that office procedures are altered to prevent further complaints as necessary, and training is reinforced in common complaint areas.

The final major responsibility, the sanction process, functions in concert with the complaint process. Although HIPAA does not specify the nature of the sanctions, the organization must apply reasonable sanctions that are consistent with the seriousness of the violations. It must be noted, however, that a violation of HIPAA can also provoke civil and criminal penalties; therefore, all violations and sanctions must be taken seriously. Sanctions can include termination of an offending employee and additional penalties. It is absolutely necessary that the manager retain documentation establishing that the employee was trained and did attend awareness meetings. It is unreasonable to expect the employees to observe HIPAA regulations if they have not been adequately trained. A sample of a form for documenting training appears as Exhibit 5.

In many organizations, HIPAA training documentation is kept with general employee training records and is maintained by the HR department. No matter who maintains the records, however, the HIPAA privacy and security officers remain accountable for training employees on the HIPAA Privacy and Security Rules.

Exhibit 5

HIPAA Training Record

Name: _____

Employee identification number: _____

Department: _____

Employment start date: _____

Date	Training Topic	Comments
_____	_____	_____
_____	_____	_____
_____	_____	_____

Keeping Up with HIPAA

With six of the eleven rules of HIPAA implemented, healthcare managers have much to do. As seen with HITECH and its influence the HIPAA Privacy and Security Rules, while managers await the next five rules, they must also remain current with the original six. When HIPAA is essentially up and running in the organization, this task of keeping up to date becomes less daunting. Managers are encouraged to attend conferences, join professional associations, read the literature, and foster awareness of HIPAA throughout their organizations.

Questions for Review and Discussion

1. Under HIPAA are patients allowed to alter their health information records? If so, how must this be done?
2. Why is documentation of HIPAA training necessary?
3. Define the term "business associate" and describe how and by whom the activities of such associates are controlled.
4. What are the circumstances that primarily govern anyone's access to a patient's personal medical information?
5. What is the purpose of the Health Information Technology Economic and Clinical Health Act (HITECH) implemented February 17, 2010?
6. What do you believe have been the biggest objections to HIPAA voiced by managers and administrators?
7. So far, what seem to have been the greatest visible effects of HIPAA?
8. Describe the form or forms in which a covered organization must maintain its HIPAA records.
9. What do you consider to be the primary reasons for the enactment of HIPAA?
10. What is the general legal attitude toward the absence of documentation needed to resolve a complaint or respond to a challenge?

References

1. Mossman, V. S. (2006). Recap of HIPAA information sessions and guidelines. *Action Newsletter, American College Health Association, 46*(1).
2. 45 CFR 160.103. Standards for Privacy of Individually Identifiable Health Information. US Department of Health and Human Services, Office for Civil Rights. (2000, December 28).
3. 45 CFR 164.520(b)(3). Health Insurance Reform: Security Standards, Final Rule. US Department of Health and Human Services, Office for Civil Rights. (2003, February 20).

Informed Consent and Patient Rights: Patient Self-Determination

Dawn M. Oetjen, PhD, *Program Director, MS, Health Services Administration, Department of Health Management and Informatics, College of Health & Public Affairs, University of Central Florida, Orlando, Florida*

Reid M. Oetjen, PhD, *Program Director, Executive MS, Health Services Administration, Department of Health Management and Informatics, College of Health & Public Affairs, University of Central Florida, Orlando, Florida*

Chapter Objectives

- Review the history and evolution of informed consent and convey its importance in the present-day provision of health care.
- Introduce and review the various elements and components of informed consent and the reasons for their existence.
- Review the types of informed consent and the rules and guidelines for determining who may provide consent.
- Address patient rights and responsibilities as set forth in the Patient Bill of Rights.
- Develop an understanding of the present-day uses of privacy and confidentiality and how these apply to individuals and to their personal medical information.

Informed Consent

Patients and their families are becoming increasingly more responsible as partners in their health care. One significant dimension of this expanded responsibility involves the use of informed consent.

As it is generally used, informed consent refers to both a legal document and the conditions addressed in that document. Recognized in all 50 states, informed consent conveys an individual's consent to a surgical or medical procedure or participation in a clinical study. It is based upon a clear appreciation and understanding of the facts, implications, and potential consequences of an action. The informed consent process is based on the moral and legal premise of patient autonomy, whereby patients have the right to make decisions about their health and medical conditions, and physicians have a duty to involve patients in decisions regarding their health care.

History

Informed consent, whether as a concept or the term itself, has often been traced back to the Nuremberg Trials during which 26 Nazi physicians were tried for research atrocities performed on prisoners of war and others. Resulting from these trials was the Nuremberg Code, the first recognized international code governing medical research. One of the primary foci of this chapter is to illuminate the requirement of *voluntary informed consent* of the human subject, thereby protecting the right of the individual to control his or her own body. This code also recognizes that risk must be weighed against the expected benefit, that unnecessary pain and suffering must be avoided, and that doctors should avoid actions that injure human patients.

The principles established by this code of medical practice have now been extended into general codes of medical ethics. Yet, as a code written in response to crimes against humanity, and, more specifically, written with regard to nontherapeutic human-subject research, the Nuremberg Code had little impact on the actual practice of therapeutic clinical research at the time of its writing, and, in fact, did not mention specifically informed consent.[1, 2]

More correctly, the term informed consent was believed by many to have been used first by Gebhard in a 1957 malpractice case, *Salgo v. Leland Stanford, Jr., the University Board of Trustees*.[3–5] In this case, the California Supreme Court stated that no patient can submit to a medical intervention without having given prior "informed consent." This ruling has been referenced for more than 45 years by medical historians, legal analysts, and medical ethicists as the event from which the term first originated.[2]

However, in 1995, the final report of the President's Advisory Committee on Human Radiation Experiments provided an even earlier history of the concept.[6] Through the committee's extensive research of archival materials from the Atomic Energy Commission (AEC), a letter was discovered, written in 1947 by the general manager of the newly formed AEC to a clinical investigator on an obscure and new requirement regarding the need for "informed consent." The letter was written specifically in response to the investigator's request to allow the declassification of data from government-sponsored radiation research on cancer patients, so that it might be reported and published by the investigator. As exemplified in the letter, the newly formed AEC clearly had significant concerns about potential litigation problems because of the use of seemingly vulnerable cancer patients as research subjects without any documentation of consent.[2]

Elements of Full Informed Consent

Although the specific definition of informed consent may vary from state to state, the elements of full informed consent are generally consistent. The physician must discuss with the individual involved the following elements:

- The individual's diagnosis (if known) and nature of the decision or proposed treatment or procedure;
- The benefits and risks of the decision or proposed treatment or procedure;
- Alternative decisions, treatments, or procedures;
- The benefits and risks of these alternatives;
- The benefits and risks of not receiving or undergoing any treatment or procedure;
- An opportunity for questions by individual and time for reflection;
- An assessment of patient understanding; and
- Acceptance (or refusal) of decision, treatment, procedure, or alternatives.

Components of Informed Consent

Informed consent involves more than simply getting a patient to sign a written consent form that outlines the aforementioned elements. It is a two-way communication process between an individual and physician that results in the individual's authorization or agreement to undergo a specific medical intervention.

There are four components of informed consent. First, in order to give informed consent, the individual concerned must have the capacity or ability to make the decision. Impairments to reasoning and judgment that would make it impossible to provide informed consent include conditions such as severe mental retardation, severe mental illness, intoxication, severe sleep deprivation, Alzheimer's disease, or being in a coma or persistent vegetative state (PVS).

Second, the individual must be in possession of all relevant facts at the time consent is given. There must be adequate disclosure of information. The law requires that a reasonable physician–patient standard be applied when determining how much information is considered adequate. There are three approaches to making this decision: (1) providing what the typical physician would say about the decision, treatment, or procedure (the reasonable physician standard); (2) providing what the average patient would say about the decision, treatment, or procedure (the reasonable patient standard); and (3) providing what this individual patient would need to know and understand to make an informed decision (the subjective standard).[7]

Third, the individual must comprehend the relevant information. The physician must evaluate whether or not the individual has understood what has been said, must ascertain that the risks have been accepted, and that the individual is giving consent to proceed with the decision, treatment, or procedure with full knowledge and forethought.[7] The individual shares this responsibility with the physician in that the physician may not realize that some items discussed were not understood until the individual asks questions or asks for more information.

And, fourth, individuals must voluntarily grant consent, without coercion or duress. Freedom of choice must exist, including the choice to go against medical advice and do nothing. To ensure that consent is voluntary, physicians should make clear to the individuals involved that they are actively participating in the decision and not simply signing a form.

Through addressing these four requirements, the following necessary conditions for informed consent are satisfied: (1) that the individual's decision is voluntary; (2) that the decision is made with an appropriate understanding of the circumstances; and (3) that the patient's choice is deliberate and that the patient has carefully considered all of the expected benefits, burdens, risks, and reasonable alternatives.

Types of Consent

Not all situations require that informed consent be given. For example, although listening to respirations through a stethoscope could be considered a treatment or procedure, it is not likely that a physician and patient would have a lengthy discussion about the risks and benefits of this care. This nonwritten consent that occurs when an individual cooperates with a particular action initiated by a physician is termed implied (indirect or deemed) consent.

Expressed (explicit or direct) consent, in oral or written form, should be obtained when the treatment or procedure is likely to be more than mildly painful or when it carries appreciable risk. If an individual were to agree to a surgical procedure, the physician would have the individual sign an expressed consent form.

Who Gives Consent?

Adults

Generally, adults, 18 years of age or older with decision-making capacity, are expected to make choices regarding their own treatment. Adults have decision-making capacity if they (1) have not been declared incompetent by the courts, and (2) are capable of evaluating alternatives, understanding the consequences of the alternatives, and selecting and acting accordingly. These decisions, made by competent adults, are usually outlined in advance directives, such as living wills. A surrogate decision maker or healthcare proxy may also be appointed by the individual to speak on their behalf. These advance directives and proxies are effective even if the individual becomes incapacitated.

If no advance directive exists and an individual is determined to be incapacitated or incompetent to make healthcare decisions, there is a specific hierarchy of appropriate decision makers defined by state law. In the absence of a state statute, the most widely accepted order of priority of close family is spouse, adult children, parents, adult siblings, and others. When there is more than one close family member or other person with knowledge of the individual's wishes, a family conference might be held to achieve consensus.[8] When consensus is not possible, or if there is no appropriate decision maker available, the physicians are expected to act in the best interest of the individual until a surrogate can be appointed. A court-appointed surrogate or proxy can also be appointed by a judge if requested by a physician, family member, friend, or an organization. This process varies from state to state.

Minors

If the individual is a minor, that is, younger than 18 years of age, the concept of informed consent has little direct application. Although minors may have appropriate decision-making capacity, they usually do not have the legal empowerment to give informed consent. Therefore, parents or other surrogate decision makers may give informed consent for diagnosis and treatment of a minor, preferably with the assent of the minor whenever possible. Most states also have laws that designate some minors as emancipated and entitled to the full rights of adults. These exceptions include minors who are: (1) self-supporting or not living in their parent's home; (2) married; (3) pregnant or a parent; (4) in the military; or (5) declared emancipated by a court. Most states also give decision-making authority to otherwise "mature minors" (unemancipated minors with decision-making capacity) who are seeking treatment for certain medical conditions, such as drug or alcohol abuse, pregnancy, or sexually transmitted diseases.[9]

No matter who is appointed to make the decision, the goal should remain the same: to make the decision that the individual would want if able to express it, and, if this is not known, to make the decision that is in the best interest of the individual.

When Consent Requirements Do Not Apply

An individual's consent should only be presumed, rather than obtained, in emergency situations when the individual is unconscious or incompetent and no surrogate decision maker is available. This privilege to proceed in emergency situations is extended to physicians because inaction at this time could cause greater harm to the patient and would be contrary to good medical practice; however, every effort should be made to document the urgent medical need for the procedure prior to proceeding.[10]

Managerial Implications

The process of obtaining informed consent, prevalent throughout healthcare facilities, is fraught with confusion, gaps, miscommunication, and potential for lawsuits. Most consent forms have been drafted by attorneys largely for attorneys and are difficult for many readers because of their complex legal terminology. In fact, researchers report that some 44% of patients who sign consent forms do not fully understand the exact nature of the procedure to be performed, and almost 70% did not read or understand the information on the form.[11]

Communicating the risks, benefits, and alternatives of procedures is often as challenging for the clinician as understanding is for the patient. Further complicating the matter is the fact that most physicians receive little or no training in how to communicate this information to their patients.[12] A prudent healthcare manager is advised to modify the informed consent process and offer one that is simplified yet complete, so there can be no doubt whether the patient has been informed.

For successful informed consent, there must be shared decision making such that patients are actively involved with their clinicians in reaching healthcare decisions. If this does not occur, interventions might be provided to patients who would not normally choose them and withheld from those who would.[13] Thus, it is critical that clinical personnel engage patients in a discussion about the nature and scope of the procedure and encourage patients to be active and informed participants in the process.[14] Healthcare organizations and clinicians are encouraged to make a commitment to transparency with patients about risks, benefits, and alternatives, whether good or bad.

One method of doing so involves creating forms that utilize simple language, translated as necessary into the primary language of the patient. This sort of consent form should be used as a guide for the essential discussion between physician and patient. The National Quality Forum (NQF) suggests that healthcare organizations then ask patients or their surrogates to repeat what has been told to them in their own words to ensure that the elements of the informed consent discussion are understood.

When working with patients exhibiting weak proficiency in English, a low literacy level, or problems with vision or hearing, appropriate accommodations should be made.[14] Healthcare organizations should provide patients with the necessary assistance; the costs of doing so are inconsequential when considered relative to the legal implications of failing to do so. Additionally, clinicians need to be sensitive to patients' cultural beliefs and practices in order to avoid misunderstandings.

Patients' Rights and Responsibilities

In addition to informed consent, there are numerous other patient rights and responsibilities. These are articulated in the *Consumer Bill of Rights and Responsibilities* that was adopted by the US Advisory Commission on Consumer Protection and

Quality in the Health Care Industry in 1988. It is also known as the *Patient Bill of Rights* and was created with the intent of reaching three major goals: (1) to help patients feel more confident in the US healthcare system by ensuring that the system is fair and that it works to meet patients' needs, gives patients a way to address any problems they may have, and encourages patients to take an active role in staying or getting healthy; (2) to stress the importance of a strong relationship between patients and their healthcare providers; and (3) to stress the key role patients play in staying healthy by laying out rights and responsibilities for all patients and healthcare providers. These rights and responsibilities include: information disclosure, choice of providers and plans, access to emergency services, participation in treatment decisions, respect and nondiscrimination, privacy and confidentiality of health information, and complaints and appeals.[15]

Information Disclosure

In addition to being well-informed about the treatment options available to them, individuals have the right to accurately and easily understand information about their health plans along with the healthcare professionals and facilities that are available to choose from or those who are already their care providers. Information regarding health care can be quite complex and often cannot be explained to or understood by an individual at any literacy level. Whenever possible, this information should be clearly and concisely written in a manner that can be understood by all, or at a maximum, a 4th grade level of reading. While the average literacy level of Americans is typically higher (at about a 7th or 8th grade reading level), the terminology used in health care is more complex and intimidating to readers; therefore, writing at a lower level is less likely to hinder comprehension.

Additionally, the United States is a melting pot of many cultures, each with its own language and customs. Facilities should ensure that individuals receive from all staff members effective, understandable, and respectful care that is provided in a manner compatible with cultural health beliefs and practices and in the individual's preferred language. Language assistance services, including bilingual staff and interpreter services, should be offered at no cost to individuals with limited English proficiency at all points of contact in a timely manner and during all hours of operation. Facilities should also make available easily understood health-related materials and post signage in the languages of the commonly encountered groups and/or groups represented in the service area.[16]

Choice of Providers and Plans

With the continually rising cost of health care and the frequently encountered barriers to accessing care, individuals deserve the opportunity to exercise choice regarding treatment providers and options. The concept of choice is deeply ingrained in American consumers and can be traced back to the guarantees provided in the

US Constitution. Thus, individuals should have both the expectation and the right to personally choose properly trained and credentialed healthcare providers who can furnish high quality health care when it is needed. This right to choose one's own healthcare facilities, providers, and health plans is considered sacred by many, and any threat can quickly mobilize consumers to fight to retain their right.

Access to Emergency Services

Individuals have the right to access emergency healthcare services when and where the need arises. Health plans use a "prudent layperson" standard in determining eligibility for coverage of emergency services. Coverage of emergency department services must be available without authorization if there is reason to believe an individual's life is in danger or that the person would be seriously injured or disabled without immediate care. Individuals have the right to be screened and stabilized using emergency services and should be able to use these services whenever and wherever needed, without having to wait for authorization and without financial penalty.

Participation in Treatment Decisions

As discussed in the previous section, individuals have the right to know their treatment options and to take part in decisions about their care. For persons who may be incompetent or unable to make these decisions, parents, guardians, family members, or others selected by the individual can represent them.

Additionally, individuals have the right to refuse treatment. Except for legally authorized involuntary treatment, persons who are legally competent to make medical decisions and who are judged by healthcare providers to have decision-making capacity have the legal and moral right to refuse any and all treatment. This is true even if the individual chooses to use poor judgment that may result in serious disability or even death.

Individuals also have the right to refuse information or to ask that only minimal information be given to them and, instead, rely on the health provider to make decisions regarding their care. The healthcare provider should make sure that the individual has clearly expressed this refusal in writing.

Respect and Nondiscrimination

Individuals have a right to considerate, nondiscriminatory, and respectful care from healthcare providers and health plan representatives at all times and under all circumstances. Individuals must not be discriminated against in the delivery of healthcare services, consistent with the benefits covered in their policy or as required by law. Individuals who are eligible for coverage under the terms and conditions of a health plan or program or as required by law also must not be discriminated against in marketing and enrollment practices based on race, ethnicity, national origin, religion, sex, age, mental or physical disability, sexual orientation, genetic information, or source of payment. This environment of mutual respect is essential to maintaining a quality healthcare system.[15]

Privacy and Confidentiality of Health Information

The Health Insurance Portability and Accountability Act (HIPAA) Privacy Rule provides federal guidelines to protect the confidentiality of identifiable medical information (see Chapter 2). It also gives individuals more control over and knowledge regarding the persons or entities who will be using their medical information and for what purposes. Also, the HIPAA Patient Safety Rule protects identifiable information from being used to analyze patient safety events and improve patient safety (see Chapter 2 for additional information concerning HIPAA).

Privacy

Privacy and confidentiality are terms that are often used interchangeably; however, in actuality, they are largely separate concepts. Privacy is an individual's right to control the access of oneself by others. Individuals decide with whom, when, and where to share their personal information. For example, individuals may not want to be seen entering places that might stigmatize them, or they may not want to share certain diagnoses with their employers.

To ensure that an individual's privacy is not breached, there are certain measures that can be taken by healthcare organizations. These measures include the following: (1) Discussions and consultations containing identifiable patient information should take place in areas that afford discretion and confidentiality, and never in elevators, hallways, cafeterias, or other areas where nonmedical staff may be present. (2) Common courtesies, such as knocking on doors before entering and closing bedside curtains prior to initiating physical exams should be extended to all individuals. (3) Discretion should be observed when leaving messages on answering machines or when faxing information. (4) Individuals should be informed of all personnel present and involved in their care, including observers, interns, and medical students.

Confidentiality

Privacy generally concerns people, whether singly or in concert. Confidentiality, however, concerns information. Today's enlightened outlook concerning confidentiality conveys the belief that information about an individual should be controllable by that individual, and that the individual has the right to specify what personal information can be communicated and to whom it can be communicated. Thus, policies concerning information handling are placed before all who enter the healthcare system, and individuals must designate who, if anyone other than the providers involved in their care, is entitled to access to that information.

Privacy and confidentiality certainly overlap to some extent, especially in situations in which breaching confidentiality may also entail invading privacy. Consider the simplest of examples: You are hospitalized in a unit that is identified with a particular kind of medical problem. You want no one to know where you are and you want no one to visit you. But someone "slips" and advises an intended visitor where you are; the room and unit identification set you up for a violation of privacy because others now know where you are, and a breach of confidentiality has occurred because one can infer from the information received what your medical issue might be as well as knowing you are indeed hospitalized. Thus, privacy and confidentiality, though separable concepts, are frequently found hand-in-hand.

Complaints and Appeals

You have the right to a fair, fast, and objective review of any complaint you have against your health plan, hospitals, doctors, or other healthcare personnel. This includes complaints about waiting times, hours of operation, the actions of healthcare personnel, and the adequacy of healthcare facilities.

In a healthcare system that protects consumers' rights, it is reasonable to expect and to encourage consumers to assume reasonable responsibilities. Greater individual involvement by consumers in their care increases the likelihood of achieving the best outcomes and helps support a quality improvement and, cost-conscious environment.

The individual as a consumer can make a significant contribution in several key areas, such as by:

- Maximizing healthy habits (e.g., exercising, not smoking, and following a healthy diet);
- Becoming involved in care decisions;
- Working collaboratively with providers in developing and carrying out agreed-upon treatment plans;
- Disclosing relevant information and clearly communicating wants and needs;
- Using available disputed-claims processes when there is disagreement between individual and health plan (the process is described in plan brochures);
- Becoming knowledgeable of coverage and health plan options, including covered benefits, limitations and exclusions, rules regarding use of network providers, coverage and referral rules, appropriate processes to secure additional information, and process to appeal coverage decisions (this information is in plan brochures);
- Showing respect for other patients and for healthcare workers;
- Making a good-faith effort to meet financial obligations; and
- Reporting wrongdoing and fraud to appropriate resources or legal authorities.

Questions for Review and Discussion

1. In what ways have people not always had complete control over their own health care?
2. What do you believe is the "moral and legal premise of patient autonomy?"
3. In what ways are the patients of today being encouraged to take more responsibility for their own care?
4. Who may automatically access your personal health information without your signed permission?
5. It is understood that in its use in this chapter, consent means the granting of permission to deliver some form of care to the individual, but what makes it *informed* consent?
6. Explain in your own words the objectives of the Patient Bill of Rights.
7. What courses of action are available if an individual does not or is in no position to grant consent for medical care?
8. What is the primary purpose of an advance directive?
9. Explain in detail the differences between an advance directive and a health-care proxy.
10. What are the requirements that must be fulfilled for informed consent to be legal and valid?

References

1. Faden, R. R., Beauchamp, T. L., & King, N. M. P. (1986). *A history and theory of informed consent*. New York, NY: Oxford University Press.
2. Daugherty, C. K. (1999, May). Impact of therapeutic research on informed consent and the ethics of clinical trials: A medical oncology perspective. *Journal of Clinical Oncology*, *17*(5), 1601.
3. Salgo v. Leland Stanford, Jr., the University Board of Trustees, 317 P 2nd 170 (1957).
4. Katz, J. (1984). *The silent world of doctor and patient*. New York: The Free Press.
5. P. G. Gebhard, 69, developer of the term "informed consent" [obituary]. (1997, August 26). *The New York Times*.
6. Advisory Committee on Human Radiation Experiments. (1996). *The human radiation experiments* (pp. 46–67). New York: Oxford University Press.
7. Informed consent. (Eds.). (2005). In J. Lehman & S. Phelps (Eds.), *West's encyclopedia of American law*. Detroit: Thomson Gale.
8. Miller, R. D. (2006). *Problems in health care law*. Sudbury, MA: Jones and Bartlett Publishers.
9. American Academy of Pediatrics, Committee on Bioethics. (1995, February). Informed consent, parental permission, and assent in pediatric practice. *Pediatrics*, *95*(2), 314–317.
10. Pozgar, G. (2010). *Legal and ethical issues for health professionals*. Sudbury, MA: Jones and Bartlett Publishers.

11. National Quality Forum. (2005). *Implementing a national voluntary consensus standard for informed consent. A user's guide for healthcare professionals.* Washington, DC: Author. Available at: http://www.qualityforum.org/Publications/2005/09/Implementing_a_National_ Voluntary_Consensus_Standard_for_Informed_Consent__A_User%E2%80%99s_Guide_ for_Healthcare_Professionals.aspx. Accessed June 29, 2010.

12. Schwartz, L. M., Woloshin, S., & Welch, H. G. (1999). Risk communication in clinical practice: Putting cancer into context. *Journal of the National Cancer Institute, 1999*(25), 124–133.

13. Sepucha, K. R., Fowler, F. J., & Mulley, A. G. (2004, October 7). Policy support for patient-centered care: The need for measurable improvements in decision quality. *Health Affairs.*

14. The Joint Commission. (2009). *Patient safety essentials for health care* (5th ed.). Oak Brook Terrace, IL: Joint Commission Resources.

15. President's Advisory Commission on Consumer protection and Quality in the Health Care Industry. (1998). *Consumer Bill of Rights and Responsibilities.* Available at: http://govinfo .library.unt.edu/hcquality/cborr. Accessed November 23, 2009.

16. The Office of Minority Health. (2007*). National Standards on Culturally and Linguistically Appropriate Services (CLAS).* Available at: http://minorityhealth.hhs.gov/templates/browse .aspx?lvl=2&lvlID=15. Accessed November 17, 2009.

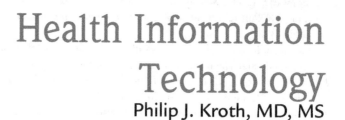

Health Information Technology

Philip J. Kroth, MD, MS

This chapter outlines major historical developments in the evolution of health information technology and discusses government initiatives to support its implementation. It highlights both benefits and challenges of using this new technology and progress in implementation to date.

Historical Overview

Applying modern information technology (IT) to the health care system to improve its quality and reduce its costs is not new. On April 27, 2004, President Bush created the Office of the National Coordinator for Health Information Technology (ONCHIT or "the ONC") by Executive Order as the first step to create the Nationwide Health Network.[1] On February 17, 2009, President Obama signed the American Recovery and Reinvestment Act (ARRA) that designated $20.8 billion through the Medicare and Medicaid reimbursement systems to incentivize physicians and health care organizations to adopt and achieve "Meaningful Use" of electronic health records (EHRs).[2]

These programs are the latest in a long history of government health information technology (HIT) initiatives. One of the earliest government inquiries into the potential benefits of HIT occurred in the Kennedy Administration in the early 1960s. A report from the

President's Science Advisory Committee, "Some New Technologies and their Promise for the Life Sciences," was optimistic about the benefits HIT would bring to biomedical research and the health care system. Ironically, the report written a half century ago is still relevant to current HIT issues:

> The application of computer technology to the recording, storage, and analysis of data collected in the course of observing and treating large numbers of ill people promises to advance our understanding of the cause, course, and control of disease. The need for a general-purpose health information technology stems in large part from increasingly rapid changes in the pattern of illness in the United States and from equally significant changes in the way medicine is practiced. The acute infectious diseases from which the patient either recovered or died have largely given place to chronic disorders which run an extremely variable course dependent on many factors both in the environment and within the patient himself. . . . Within any sizable community there are numerous administrative organizations charged with providing health services. It is not uncommon for a single patient to be cared for by a large number of agencies in a single city, and workers in any one agency usually cannot find out about the activities of others; sometimes they even fail to learn that other agencies are active at all. . . . Modern data-processing techniques make it possible to assemble all the necessary information about all the patients in a given geographical or administrative area in one place with rapid access for all authorized health and welfare agencies. Such a system would produce an immediate and highly significant improvement in medical care with a simultaneous reduction in direct dollar costs of manual record processing and an even greater economy in professional time now wasted in duplicating tests and procedures.[3]

To date, despite a half century of government programs and technological advancement, the best and most current scientific evidence indicates that the benefits of HIT on the quality and cost of health care are at best, mixed.[4] This chapter will explore the history of how HIT has evolved, the imprint HIT has made on the current health care system, and speculate about how HIT will likely influence the future of health care and the health care system as a whole.

Using computers to improve health care in many ways parallels the development of modern IT. The late 1960s and early 1970s saw several pioneering efforts at a small number of universities to apply IT to various aspects of the health care delivery process. Early systems were not the web-based, interactive systems of today but were usually a hybrid of computer and paper integrated into a clinical work process. One early example was a system at

Indiana University where a small army of data entry clerks manually entered data into a computer on key parts of all patients' medical records.

The night before a patient's clinic appointment, a one-page, paper encounter form was printed for the appointment listing the patients' name, record number, medical problem list (i.e., the known diagnoses and medical problems), medication list, medication allergies, and suggestions based on the data in the computer system. A suggestion was printed on the list when the computer software detected any of 290 agreed-upon patient care protocols or conditions defined by rules applied to the computer's database. When a physician saw the patient in the clinic, they would handwrite encounter notes on the appropriate section of the paper encounter form and manually annotate the computer-printed problem list, medication list, and other items. The next day, a team of data entry clerks would review all encounter forms and update the computer data to reflect the physician's orders and updates to the patient's condition. The paper form would then be filed to the patient's chart. The Indiana group conducted a study demonstrating a 29% improvement in adherence to agreed-upon treatment protocols in the group of physicians who received the computer "suggestions" for recommended treatment protocols on the encounter forms versus those who did not.[5] With the introduction of the IBM PC in the late 1970s and early 1980s, paper forms were mostly eliminated and physicians began interacting with the patient's EHR in real time on the video screen. Similar experimental systems were designed and built during the same time period at a number of other U.S. universities, including The University of Pittsburgh,[6] The University of Utah,[7,8] Vanderbilt University,[9,10] Duke,[11] and Harvard University/Massachusetts General Hospital.[12] These early systems were custom designed, built, and maintained by in-house dedicated teams of computer programmers and systems engineers. Because of the custom designs, the unique work process that existed at each institution, and the advanced nature of these early systems, they were not portable and could not be transplanted to other institutions without extensive software design rework. More importantly, because each of these early systems had a unique design, they were incapable of electronically transferring any of the patients' records to any other system. Despite these limitations, the pioneering works done with these early systems laid the foundation for modern EHR design.

It was not until the 1990s that commercially produced comprehensive EHR systems were marketed and sold to health care institutions in high volume. These commercially produced systems allowed hospitals to implement EHRs without the prohibitive expenses of building custom systems. Instead, hospitals could buy an "off the shelf" system that although not completely customized to institutional work flows, could be configured to meet most of their perceived HIT institutional needs. However, as with the pioneering EHR systems at academic institutions, the "off the shelf," commercially produced EHRs of today still require extensive configuration to accommodate the unique and varying work processes at each institution. The configuration differences between institutions are often so significant that even institutions with the same commercial EHR systems cannot electronically exchange patients' records without customized software. The ONC Website reports that there are a total of 2,648 certified ambulatory EHR products and a total of 878 inpatient products currently on the Certified HIT Product List.[13] While many of these are merely different versions of the same software, there are at least 200 unique systems. None of these systems is designed to interface with each other for patient data sharing across different software platforms. Due to this lack of standardization, regional health information organizations (RHIOs) have been created to facilitate the exchange of patient data among different health care institutions to support improved patient care. RHIOs and health information exchanges (HIEs) are discussed in more detail later in this chapter.

The 2009 HITECH Act created several programs to incentivize individual physicians and health care organizations to buy, install, and adopt EHR systems in the hope that this will yield significant benefits by reducing the cost and improving the quality of care.[2] "The provisions of the HITECH Act are specifically designed to work together to provide the necessary assistance and technical support to providers, enable coordination and alignment within and among states, establish connectivity to the public health community in case of emergencies, and assure the workforce is properly trained and equipped to be meaningful users of EHRs."[14] The scope of this text does not allow detailed delineations of HITECH Act programs; however, the following brief descriptions of programs created and supported by the HITECH Act provide an overview of its comprehensive approach to HIT implementation[14]:

- Beacon Community Program to assist communities in building their HIT infrastructures and exchange capabilities

- Consumer eHealth Program to help empower Americans' access to their personal health information and use this as a tool to gain more control over their health
- State Health Information Exchange Cooperative Agreement Program to support states in establishing HIE capability among health care providers and hospitals in their jurisdictions
- HIT Exchange Program to establish regional extension centers for education and training of health providers in use of EHRs
- Strategic Health IT Advanced Research Projects to fund research advances to overcome major barriers to EHR adoption

While the HITECH Act and its funding provide a new thrust toward EHR adoption, the state of EHR technology does not allow most systems to interface with each other. Despite this large government investment and over half a century of technological development, U.S. health care system HIT still consists of a large number of disparate "siloed" systems that cannot electronically exchange patient records in an efficient and secure manner.

Historical Challenges in Implementing HIT

Figure 1 illustrates the three essential components required for successful HIT implementation.

The first essential component is the technology. Organizations often focus on this first component with the mistaken belief that merely selecting the "right" technology or the "right EHR" is the most important aspect of HIT implementation. The essential technologies needed to implement an EHR

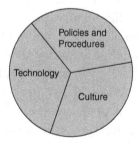

FIGURE 1 The Three Essential Components of a Successful HIT Implementation.

system are a relational database, a computer network, and computer workstation. All three technologies have existed for more than 40 years, begging the question of why adoption of HIT in the clinical environment has been so slow compared to the adoption of IT in other industries such as the airline industry's reservation system. The second component of successful implementation, work policies and procedures, makes implementing HIT systems in the clinical environment extremely challenging due to wide variations in work policies and procedures among different organizations and institutions.

An organization's policies and procedures describe and define the processes through which work is carried out. The process component is complex, because it requires HIT system implementers to fully understand all existing work processes. Many such processes are not written or formalized, having evolved over the years to accommodate the unique characteristics of a particular organization. Often existing work processes are significantly different from those officially documented or assumed to be in place, while many critical work processes are not documented at all. When a HIT system is implemented, it is common for many of the undocumented processes to become apparent for the first time.[15] Undocumented or unknown work processes have been the root cause for many HIT implementation failures.[16]

In addition, it is well known that the most significant component of HIT implementation is the institutional and organizational culture—what people are willing to do.[17] This is the most critical, least studied, and least understood of the HIT implementation components.[18] Ash and Bates summarized the importance of organizational culture with regard to EHR adoption[19]:

Content Removed Due To Copyright Restrictions

There is a significant publication bias in the biomedical literature against publishing on HIT implementation failures. Because of the human tendency to avoid publicizing individual's mistakes, the body of literature is strongly skewed toward successful implementations and studies. Unfortunately, this has made it difficult to study and understand causes of HIT implementation failures. A significant advance for the HIT industry as a whole would be a shift in its culture toward not only reporting HIT failures, but viewing them as valuable learning opportunities rather than events to be downplayed and forgotten.

One major example of a HIT implementation failure occurred at the prestigious Cedars-Sinai Hospital in Los Angeles, California, in 2002. After implementing a new $34 million HIT system, several hundred physicians refused to use the new system 3 months after it was turned on. Cedars-Sinai attempted to implement a new electronic medical record that changed the way physicians ordered patient treatments and tests in the hospital. Prior to implementing the new system, physicians wrote their orders on paper forms in the patients' paper charts. After new patient orders were written, physicians gave the chart to nurses or ward clerks to read and implement the orders. The new system required physicians to type orders directly into a computer workstation, where the software provided the physician with immediate feedback if they attempted to enter an order that the computer either did not understand or interpreted as a mistake. An article in the *Washington Post* reported[20]:

> A veteran physician at the prestigious Cedars-Sinai Medical Center here had been mixing up a certain drug dosage for decades. Every time he wrote the prescription for 10 times the proper amount, a nurse simply corrected it, recalled Paul Hackmeyer. The computers arrived—and when the doctor typed in his medication order, the machine barked at him and he barked back. . . . "What we discovered was that for 20 years he was writing the wrong dose."

This failure illustrates the three principal HIT implementation components described above. Technology: With physicians required to enter

---

*Reproduced from the *Journal of the American Medical Informatics Association*, "Factors and forces affecting EHR system adoption: report of a 2004 ACMI discussion," by JS Ash and DW Bates, Issue 12.1, pages 8–12, © 2005, with permission from BMJ Publishing Group Ltd.

orders directly to the computer system, time required to enter orders became dependent on the computer's ordering input format and system response time. Process: Many undocumented processes in the old system were not carried to the new system. In this example, the nurse's automatic correction of an obvious dosage error was a critical, undocumented, process step—a check on the orders' accuracy. Although the new system caught the error, the physician user in this case could no longer rely on the nurse's checking and correcting his orders. Culture: The new system required physicians to interact with a computer, which took more time than writing orders on paper forms. The new system required physicians to change the way they practiced medicine in the hospital and as is common, people dislike change. This was a significant change in physicians' work culture in which nurses had routinely checked and corrected physician orders without communicating the corrections. Physicians also had to deal with a barrage of system alerts when they were imprecise or inaccurate in entering their orders. While possibly enhancing patient safety, responding to the system alerts increased the time required for physicians to place orders.

Another historical barrier to broad implementation of HIT is the chasm between those who bear the costs of the technology and those who receive its benefits. The purchase and operation of an EHR system represent a major investment for large health care organizations and especially for small private physician groups. Not only must physician groups bear the costs of the hardware and software, but they must also support ongoing IT maintenance, staff training, and software upgrade costs. Because small practice groups often have no experience or expertise with IT issues, they also experience anxiety about making decisions necessary to convert from paper to electronic charting. While economies of scale make the marginal costs of adopting EHR technology somewhat lower for large health care organizations, these organizations often do not realize costs savings from their investment. For example, a health care system participating in a HIE may reduce the number of duplicate laboratory and imaging tests saving the patient and the payer significant expense, but the health care system may actually lose money by not receiving revenue for the duplicate tests. As with large health care systems, small practices that invest in EHR technology may not directly benefit from the technology. Patients may receive better age appropriate screening[21,22] and preventative care[23] as well as reduced duplicate testing because of physician access to HIEs and patient records from outside of the practice group or health system.[24] However, from a practice financial perspective, these factors actually may produce a significant disincentive for adopting EHRs.

The Federal Government's Response to HIT Implementation Challenges

The federal government's financial incentive programs for large health care organizations and private practices that adopt and demonstrate "meaningful use" of EHRs are an effort to bridge the chasm between costs and benefits. On April 27, 2004, President Bush created the ONCHIT or "the ONC" by Executive Order.[1] In 2009, the ONC was also tasked in the Health Information Technology for Economic and Clinical Health Act (HITECH Act)[25] to be "the principal Federal entity charged with coordination of nationwide efforts to implement and use the most advanced HIT and the electronic exchange of health information."[26] The ONC's mission is to promote the development of a nationwide HIT infrastructure, provide leadership in the development of standards, provide the certification of HIT products, coordinate HIT policy, perform strategic planning for HIT adoption and HIE, and establish the governance for the Nationwide Health Information Network. Figure 2 depicts the ONC's organizational structure.[27]

The ONC employs 191 full-time staff and operates with an annual budget of $66 million in fiscal year 2013, excluding the $20.8 billion in HITECH funding in incentive payments for physicians and health care organizations administered through the Centers for Medicare and Medicaid Services for achieving meaningful use of EHRs. In addition to these resources, the HITECH Act created a HIT Policy Committee and a HIT Standards Committee under the auspices of the Federal Advisory Committee Act. Both committees have multiple workgroups with representatives from payers, academia, and the health care industry. They address a variety of HIT-related issues including certification/adoption, governance, HIE, meaningful use, privacy and security, quality measures, implementation, and a HIT vocabulary standards committee.[28]

> The Health IT Policy Committee will make recommendations to the National Coordinator for Health IT on a policy framework for the development and adoption of a nationwide health information infrastructure, including standards for the exchange of patient medical information. The American Recovery and Reinvestment Act of 2009 (ARRA) provides that the Health IT Policy Committee shall at least make recommendations on the areas in which standards, implementation specifications, and certifications criteria are needed in eight specific areas.
>
> The Health IT Standards Committee is charged with making recommendations to the National Coordinator for Health IT on standards,

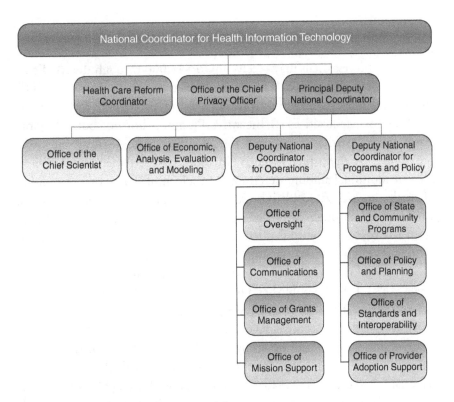

FIGURE 2 ONC Organizational Structure.
Source: Reproduced from Office of the National Coordinator for Health Information Technology Newsroom, http://www.healthit.gov/newsroom/about-onc.

implementation specifications, and certification criteria for the electronic exchange and use of health information.

As noted previously, the ONC also has funded several programs to facilitate the adoption of EHRs. Examples include training programs to increase the number of professionals with IT skills required in the health care domain. Other programs fund the development of HIE standards across multiple EHR vendor platforms. The ONC also funds annual surveys to track HIT adoption.

Meaningful Use Incentives

The $20.8 billion included in the HITECH Act created the Medicare and Medicaid EHR incentive programs for eligible professionals (individual physicians in solo or multiphysician practice groups) and hospitals as they adopt, implement, upgrade, or demonstrate meaningful use of certified EHR technology to improve patient care.[20]

Eligible professionals may receive up to $44,000 through the Medicare EHR Incentive Program and up to $63,750 through the Medicaid EHR Incentive Program. Eligible professionals may participate in either the Medicare or Medicaid EHR Incentive Programs but not both. Eligible hospitals can participate in both the Medicare and Medicaid incentive programs.[29] Each hospital incentive includes a base payment of $2 million plus an additional amount determined by a formula based on the number of discharges per year.[30,31] The Medicare Program is a 5-year program administered through the federal government while the Medicaid program is a 6-year program funded by the federal government but administered through individual states. Table 1 compares Medicare and Medicaid adoption incentive programs for eligible professionals and hospitals.[29–37] CMS also publishes a flow chart to help Eligible Professionals determine qualifications to meet program requirements.[32]

To receive EHR incentive payments, providers and hospitals must demonstrate that they are "meaningfully using" their EHRs by meeting thresholds for several specific objectives. In a partnership with the ONC, CMS has established the objectives for "meaningful use" that eligible professionals and eligible hospitals must meet in order to receive incentive payments.[38] The CMS meaningful use criteria are developed by the experts who comprise the various work groups in the ONC's Health IT Policy Committee. The level of evidence for the majority of meaningful use objectives is only at the expert opinion level. The science of HIT awaits rigorous research studies to validate the choices and designs of the meaningful use criteria.

To receive incentive payments, eligible professionals and health care organizations must meet specific meaningful use criteria in three stages. Stages 1 and 2 have been defined, but stage 3 is yet to be developed. Stage 1 includes objectives for capturing patient data and sharing data in a standardized format with patients and other health care professionals. Stage 2 includes objectives for advanced clinical processes. Stage 3 will reportedly be related to measuring and reporting clinically relevant patient outcomes.

To receive the full Medicare incentive, physicians and hospitals were required to apply for Stage 1 certification by 2012 or the maximum amount of the Medicare incentive payments decreases each year until 2015 when the Medicare incentive stops.[39] The Medicaid incentive payments for eligible professionals are higher under the Medicaid EHR

Table 1 Comparison of Medicare and Medicaid Adoption Incentive Programs for Eligible Professionals (Individual Physicians in Solo and Group Practices) and Hospitals (Including Critical Access Hospitals)[29-37]

	Medicare Program	Medicaid Program
Eligible Professionals	• Administered by CMS • $44,000 Maximum per physician (over 5-year period) • 90% or more of practice must be outpatient based • Cannot participate in Medicaid Program if enrolled in Medicare Program • Must apply for Stage 1 Meaningful Use by 2012 to obtain the maximum incentive • Medicare imposes payment penalty on those failing to demonstrate Meaningful Use by 2015	• Administered by State Medicaid Agency • $63,750 Maximum per physician participate (over 5 years) • Must have ≤30% Medicaid patient volume or ≤20% Medicaid patient volume and be a pediatrician or practice predominantly in a Federally Qualified Health Center or Rural Health Clinic and have ≤30% patient volume attributable to needy individuals • ≤90% of practice must be outpatient based • Cannot participate in Medicare Program if enrolled in Medicaid Program • Can begin to certify for Meaningful Use by 2016 and still receive full incentive • Non-participants exempt from Medicaid payment reductions
Hospitals (including Critical Access Hospitals)	• Administered by CMS • Can begin receiving incentive FY 2011 to FY 2015, but payments will decrease for hospitals that start receiving payments in FY 2014 and later • Medicare and Medicaid Program eligible	• Administered by State Medicaid Agency • Acute care hospitals (including critical access and cancer hospitals) with at least 10% Medicaid patient volume are eligible • Children's hospitals are eligible regardless of their Medicaid volume

- Must apply for Stage 1 Meaningful Use by FY 2013 to receive maximum incentive
- Hospitals that do not successfully demonstrate Meaningful Use will be subject to Medicare payment penalties beginning in FY 2015
- Incentive payments are based on several factors, beginning with a $2 million base payment

- Can apply for both Medicare and Medicaid Programs
- Incentive payments are based on a number of factors, beginning with a $2 million base payment

Source: Centers for Medicare and Medicaid Services. Eligible Hospital Information. 2012; http://www.cms.gov/Regulations-and-Guidance/Legislation/EHRIncentivePrograms/Eligible_Hospital_Information.html. Accessed October 30, 2012; Centers for Medicare and Medicaid Services. EHR Incentive Program for Medicare Hospitals. 2012; http://www.cms.gov/Outreach-and-Education/Medicare-Learning-Network-MLN/MLNProducts/downloads/EHR_TipSheet_Medicare_Hosp.pdf. Accessed October 30, 2012; Centers for Medicare and Medicaid Services. Medicaid Hospital Incentive Payments Calculations. 2012; http://www.cms.gov/Outreach-and-Education/Medicare-Learning-Network-MLN/MLNProducts/downloads/Medicaid_Hosp_Incentive_Payments_Tip_Sheets.pdf. Accessed October 30, 2012; Centers for Medicare and Medicaid Services. Flow Chart to Help Eligible Professionals (EP) Determine Eligibility for the Medicare and Medicaid Electronic Health Record (EHR) Incentive Programs. 2012; https://www.cms.gov/Regulations-and-Guidance/Legislation/EHRIncentivePrograms/downloads/eligibility_flow_chart.pdf. Accessed December 21, 2012; Centers for Medicare and Medicaid Services. EHR Incentive Programs. 2012; http://www.cms.gov/Regulations-and-Guidance/Legislation/EHRIncentivePrograms/index.html?redirect=/ehrincentiveprograms/. Accessed September 24, 2012; Centers for Medicare and Medicaid Services. Medicare Electronic Health Record Incentive Program for Eligible Professionals. 2012; http://www.cms.gov/Outreach-and-Education/Medicare-Learning-Network-MLN/MLNProducts/Downloads/CMS_eHR_Tip_Sheet.pdf. Accessed December 22, 2012; Centers for Medicare and Medicaid Services. An Introduction to the Medicaid EHR Incentive Program for Eligible Professionals. 2012; http://www.cms.gov/Regulations-and-Guidance/Legislation/EHRIncentivePrograms/Downloads/EHR_Medicaid_Guide_Remediated_2012.pdf. Accessed December 22, 2012; Centers for Medicare and Medicaid Services. An Introduction to the Medicare EHR Incentive Program for Eligible Professionals. 2012; http://www.cms.gov/Regulations-and-Guidance/Legislation/EHRIncentivePrograms/Downloads/Beginners_Guide.pdf. Accessed December 22, 2012; Centers for Medicare and Medicaid Services. Medicaid Electronic Health Record Incentive Payments for Eligible Professionals. 2012; http://www.cms.gov/Outreach-and-Education/Medicare-Learning-Network-MLN/MLNProducts/Downloads/EHRIP_Eligible_Professionals_Tip_Sheet.pdf. Accessed December 22, 2012.

Incentive Program. Unlike the Medicare EHR Incentive Program, the Medicaid EHR Incentive Program does not penalize those who begin to certify meaningful use after 2012. In fact, an eligible professional can begin to certify meaningful use in the Medicaid Program as late as 2016 and still receive the same total incentive payment as those who began to certify in 2011. Those eligible professionals who begin to certify under the Medicaid Program after 2016 will receive no incentive. Regardless of which of the two programs certifies an eligible professional, beginning in 2015, Medicare will impose payment penalties upon providers who fail to demonstrate meaningful use. Table 2 summarizes the timetable for meaningful use criteria implementation.[40]

Detailed information on the Meaningful Use requirements for Stage 1 is available for eligible professionals[41] and eligible hospitals.[42] Some examples of meaningful use requirements for Stage 1 for Eligible Professionals include:

- CPOE
- Drug–Drug Interaction and Drug–Allergy Checking
- Up-to-Date Problem List of Current and Active diagnoses
- Electronic or "e-prescribing" (of at least 40% of prescriptions)

Table 2 Meaningful Use Implementation Timeline[40]

Stage 1: 2011–2012	Stage 2: 2014	Stage 3: 2016
Meaningful use criteria focus on: • Electronically capturing health information in a standardized format • Using that information to track key clinical conditions • Communicating that information for care coordination processes • Initiating the reporting of clinical quality measures and public health information • Using information to engage patients and their families in their care	Meaningful use criteria focus on: • More rigorous health information exchange (HIE) • Increased requirements for e-prescribing and incorporating lab results • Electronic transmission of patient care summaries across multiple settings • More patient-controlled data	Meaningful use criteria focus on: • Improving quality, safety, and efficiency, leading to improved health outcomes • Decision support for national high-priority conditions • Patient access to self-management tools • Access to comprehensive patient data through patient-centered HIE • Improving population health

Source: Office of the National Coordinator for Health Information Technology. Stages of Meaningful Use. http://www.healthit.gov/policy-researchers-implementers/meaningful-use; United States Department of Health and Human Services. Meaningful Use. 2012; http://www.healthit.gov/policy-researchers-implementers/meaningful-use. Accessed December 21, 2012.

- Maintaining an Active Medication List
- Record and Chart Changes in Vital Signs
- Recording Smoking Status for Patients 13 Years and Older
- Reporting Ambulatory Clinical Quality Measures to CMS and States
- Implementing Clinical Decision Support
- Providing Patients with an Electronic Copy of Their Health Information Upon Request
- Providing Clinical Summaries to Patients for Each Office Visit

Stage 1 also includes a "menu" of requirements from which physicians must achieve a total of 5. Examples of requirements include the capability to generate lists of patients by specific conditions, proactively sending reminders to patients for preventive/follow-up care, providing patients with electronic access to health information, reconciling patient medication lists, and producing summaries of records for transitions of care. Stage 2 requirements build those of Stage 1 and contain 17 required objectives and a menu of six items from which to choose three. The complete list of meaningful use objectives and metrics for individual physicians and health care organizations are available.[43,44] The list of meaningful use objectives to attain Stage 3 compliance is not yet published but scheduled for release in time for the first Stage 3 certifications in 2016.

HIT Opportunities: Improving Health Care Delivery Quality, Effectiveness, and Efficiency

With mediocre evidence to date for HIT goals to improve health care quality and reduce costs, the question looms: What is the driving force behind U.S. quest to implement HIT? The answer resides in understanding the limitations of the human brain and limited attention span. A healthy human's performance begins to measurably decrease in about 40 minutes while monitoring a continuous process.[45] These limitations explain regulations for work-time breaks for air traffic controllers, anesthesiologists, and work-hour limitations for airplane pilots and commercial truck drivers, and more recently work hour limitations for medical students and residents.[46] These regulations recognize that human performance is limited by innate biology and physiology and that fatigue degrades performance; no amount of training or willpower can overcome these biological and physiological limitations. These acknowledgements apply to health care delivery where a physician in a busy outpatient clinic or inpatient ward is much like an air traffic controller monitoring a continuous process. Patients are tightly scheduled with additional patients often "doubled-booked" at the last minute because of acute illness. Every patient must be seen and volumes of data accessed, processed, and synthesized to formulate a diagnosis and a plan of care. At the same time, the physician must document the encounter in detail, complete all required forms and insurance paperwork, respond to electronic pages and phone calls, speak with consultants, manage correspondence, and in many cases supervise midlevel providers, nursing and office staff. Stead and Hammond have shown that the amount of data accessed and used by clinicians per medical decision is increasing exponentially despite the fact that physicians' ability to cope with the higher information load remains constant.[47] The driving concept behind EHRs' potential to improve the quality and reduce the cost of health care is represented by Figure 3.[48]

The ultimate goal is to combine the intuitive strengths of humans and data retention strengths of computers to create a hybrid system that is intuitive with a tireless data processing capability. The computer reminds the physician to do what they already know how to do, and what they want to do, in a manner that makes it easy to implement. Meeting these parameters results in an efficacious computerized decision support system (CDSS). For CDSS to work, the computer system must provide the right information at the right place and at the right time. If any of these

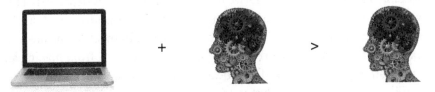

FIGURE 3 Why EHRs have Potential to Improve Quality and Reduce Costs.
Source: Adapted from Friedman CP. What informatics is and isn't. *J Am Med Inform Assoc.* 2012;0:1–3.
Computer: © *iStockphoto/Thinkstock.*
Head: © *Lightspring/Shutterstock, Inc.*

three requirements are missing, the system will tend to fail. With EHRs, the right place and time are often when the physician is entering patient orders at a computer workstation, a process termed CPOE. At this place and time, the physician's mind is focused on the patient just seen or the patient they are currently thinking about. It is also this place and time at which it is easiest for the physician to take action, such as writing new orders that result in timely follow-through for a patient's care.

For example, when a physician has completed a patient interview and examination and is using an EHR to enter e-prescriptions that will be sent securely over the internet to the patient's pharmacy, the computer can present the physician with a pop-up "reminder" that the patient is allergic to the medication being prescribed. It can also indicate that the prescribed requires at least annual kidney function monitoring and that the last record of kidney function laboratory work is more than a year old. In this event, the system can present the physician with an option to order the appropriate laboratory work or to ignore the warning with one keystroke or mouse click. Most decision support is designed with these "soft stops" or interventions that allow the physician to heed or ignore the warning as he or she believes to be most appropriate. CDSS "hard stops" do not allow physician options to ignore a warning. An example of a "hard stop" could be the use of a very expensive, broad spectrum antibiotic that by hospital policy can only be ordered by an infectious disease specialist. In this case, the CDSS would not allow the physician to order the medication but would inform them that an infectious disease consult is required to order the drug and would make ordering that consult a mouse click away. A nonmedical example of a "hard stop" is the automobile design preventing the shift of an automatic transmission out of Park and into Drive unless the brake petal is depressed. This was implemented after reports of multiple accidental injuries and deaths attributed to unanticipated automobile movements. In this, like the medical example, the decision support system prevents the operator from making an error with high probability of significant adverse consequences.

Like the first example that used a computer–paper hybrid system in the 1970s, CDSS reminds the physician to do what they already know how to do—at the right place and time and in the most convenient manner possible. Because the computer never fatigues, the reminders compensate for physicians' biological limitations and the human–computer hybrid system outperforms what either could accomplish on their own.

There are hundreds of studies and randomized controlled trials published in the peer-reviewed, biomedical literature that have demonstrated how CDSS can have a dramatic impact on improving physician performance in myriad different health care venues. CDSS similarly designed to produce pop-up warnings and recommendations to physicians have been shown to improve the ordering of age appropriate screening tests,[21,22] appropriate antibiotic prescribing for inpatients,[49] appropriate advance directive discussions with patients,[50] the use of preventative care for hospitalized patients,[21] appropriate weaning of patients from mechanical ventilators,[51] appropriate reductions of inpatient resource utilization,[52] the prevalence of Methicillin-Resistant Staph Aureus (MRSA) in a community,[53] the isolation rates of patients admitted to the hospital with drug-resistant infections,[54] the screening for sexually transmitted diseases in the Emergency Department,[55] the accurate capture and recording of patient temperatures by nurses in the inpatient setting,[56] and many others. Despite these very promising studies, until recently, most of these studies were performed at major university health care centers that had custom designed and maintained EHR software systems, maintained by local IT departments with relatively large IT support budgets compared with smaller community hospitals' budgets.[18] In 2006, Chaudhry et al. published a systematic review of 257 CDSS studies published up to 2005 that concluded 25% of the studies were from four major academic institutions that all had custom designed systems and ". . . only 9 studies evaluated multifunctional, commercially developed systems."[18] Therefore, while there are hundreds of studies demonstrating the potential for CDSS to improve the quality of care and/or reduce its costs, the appropriateness of this research to typical health care settings in other than large academic institutions is mostly unknown.

The Agency for Health Research and Quality commissioned the most systematic, rigorous, and comprehensive CDSS review of prior studies to date and published the results in 2012.[57] The systematic review analyzed 311 studies in the biomedical literature and found moderately strong evidence confirming three previously reported factors associated with successful CDSS implementation:

1. Automatic provision of decision support as part of clinician workflow
2. Provision of decision support at time and location of decision making
3. Provision of a recommendation, not just an assessment

The study also identified six additional factors that were correlated with the successful implementation of CDSS:

1. Integration with charting or order entry system to support work-flow integration
2. No need for additional clinician data entry
3. Promotion of action rather than inaction
4. Justification of decision support via provision of research evidence
5. Local user involvement in development process
6. Provision of decision support results to patients as well as providers

The study found a high strength of evidence for CDSS to improve the ordering and completing of preventative care and ordering and prescribing recommended treatments "across academic, VA, and community inpatient and ambulatory settings that had both locally and commercially developed CDSS systems."[57]

There was a moderate strength of evidence that CDSS improves appropriate ordering of clinical studies, reduces patient morbidity and cost of care, and increases health care provider satisfaction.

Studies demonstrated a low strength of evidence for CDSS impact on efficiency of the user, length of hospital stay, mortality, health-related quality of life, and "adverse events" or medical errors.

The study also pointed out some significant voids in the current biomedical literature. None of the studies addressed the impact of CDSS on health care delivery organization changes, on the number of patients seen per unit of time, on user knowledge, on system cost-effectiveness, or on physician workload.

In summary, the current cumulative evidence for the benefits of EHRs with CPOE and CDSS is mixed. Even in areas where there is a high strength of evidence such as improvement in the ordering and completing of preventative care, the effective magnitude of the improvement is small, even though statistically significant.[57]

Health Information Exchanges

Virtually none of the commercially available EHR systems available in today's market or the custom-designed systems at large academic institutions can easily exchange patients' health information with care providers outside of their institutions. Despite 50 years of efforts, patients' health information remains siloed and "It is not uncommon for a single patient to be cared for by a large number of agencies in a single city, and workers in any one agency usually cannot find out about the activities of others; sometimes they even fail to learn that other agencies are active at all."[3] Barriers to sharing patient information across multiple providers often become immediately apparent when a patient with a significant illness sees a number of different specialty physicians and attempts to coordinate the flow of information among them. Unlike other industries such as the airlines that have cooperated to create a standardized ticketing system, the health care system has been marginally successful in designing a common platform or standard to allow a patient's records to be compatible with multiple vendor systems. In addition, health domain data are orders of magnitude larger and more complex than data for ticketing in the airline industry. In addition, the Health Insurance Portability and Accountability Act (HIPAA) regulations have had a chilling effect on health care institutions' willingness to share data with other institutions because they are responsible for patient privacy and the security of patient data.

These and other factors led to development of HIEs with their corresponding administering organizations, Regional Health Information Organizations (RHIOs). RHIOs attempt to create systems, agreements, processes, and technology to manage these factors in order to facilitate the appropriate exchange of health care information between institutions and across different vendor platforms. While most all states and regions of the United States have RHIOs, the actual state of implementation and real data exchange varies widely. For example, some states have active RHIOs that are in the planning stages of establishing relationships with all key stakeholders, creating administration agreements, creating governance structures, securing funding, attempting to develop business models for sustained funding of the organization, etc. Other RHIOs have functioning HIEs where medical data are actually being exchanged between institutions and across disparate software EHR platforms. The ONC has funded many RHIOS to develop and test their national standards for HIE with the ultimate goal of creating the "Nationwide Health Information Network" that would be a network of regional networks. Despite the testing and demonstration projects to date, actively functioning HIEs exist only at regional levels.[58]

Each vendor's building toward one common standard would significantly reduce the technical complexity of data exchange. Unfortunately, vendors' products are still not being built toward one national standard to facilitate electronic HIE. Despite these limitations, there have been significant accomplishments in implementing the data and IT standards necessary to facilitate the exchange of health information among multiple EHR platforms. Today, most institutions participating in HIEs must build or configure "interface engines" that convert the institution's data format to the form used by the HIE. This is a major challenge as there is no single standard that provides sufficient specification of data formats and communication protocols. Rather, there are a number of standards that address various domains of data management. In addition, the voluminous scope of modern health care and continuous advancements in knowledge and technology make managing data in the health care domain extremely dynamic and complex.

As an example of this complexity, the Logical Observations Indexes Names and Codes (LOINC) standard was developed in the 1990s to solve a problem with an older health information communication protocol that specified how clinical data should be identified for transmission between computer systems. LOINC uniquely defines codes for information such as blood chemistry laboratory tests and clinical observations, such as patient blood pressure that can be recorded in many different formats. There are currently over 70,000 LOINC defined codes for uniquely reporting laboratory tests and clinical observations.[59] For example, there are 419 different codes for reporting blood pressure. With its unique codes for laboratory tests and clinical observations, LOINC enables computer systems receiving the data to generate exact interpretations. This is called semantic interoperability. Semantic interoperability is essential for patient record transmission from one EHR system to another so that the meaning of the critical data contained within the records is not at risk of erroneous interpretation.

Because new laboratory tests are constantly being developed and existing assays are being improved, LOINC creates and disseminates new codes so that semantic interoperability can be maintained. Old codes are not deleted from the system, ensuring that researchers using prior clinical data bases can retrieve prior results comparable with new codes. LOINC is supported by the National Library of Medicine (NLM), a division of the National Institutes of Health. The LOINC Committee publishes quarterly updates and holds bi-annual, national meetings to discuss proposed new clinical observations and laboratory tests for the assignment of new LOINC codes.

For a HIE to transfer information accurately, each EHR system must map its own internal code for each datum to a standard code to ensure that information passed from one EHR to another in the exchange is interpreted exactly the same by the receiver as it is in the sender's system. LOINC is one of the many HIT-related standards. The Systematic Nomenclature of Medicine (SNOMED) was originally developed by the College of American Pathologists (CAP) to exactly specify tissue pathologic diagnoses. The same group also developed a standard for clinical observations called SNOMED Clinical Terms (SNOMED-CT). LOINC and SNOMED-CT domain standards overlap but their design characteristics are valuable in different situations; for example, exchanging laboratory results versus coding patient problem lists within EHRs. Similar to LOINC, CAP also provides periodic updates to SNOMED-CT codes.

To keep track of the many coding standards and the terms within, the NLM built and maintains the Unified Medical Language System (UMLS), which houses a massive "metathesaurus" and a variety of tools for mapping between and discovery of over 200 biomedically related terminology standards.[60] Because LOINC, SNOMED-CT, and the 200 or so other standards are periodically updated, the UMLS is also regularly updated to keep the interstandard terminology mapping current and accurate.

Using HIEs, designated member groups of health care institutions exchange data in a standardized format using a combination of the previously described standards. This cooperation enables the access to a comprehensive clinical data set on individual patients across multiple institutions and multiple EHR vendor platforms.

There are two kinds of HIE architectures: "monolithic" and "federated."

The monolithic architecture is a design where all member institutions periodically send copies of their clinical data to one central repository where all the data reside together in one format. The advantage of this approach is that a patient's comprehensive data can be maintained in one place and in one format. However, this approach has several disadvantages. First, the frequency with which members contribute and update copies of institutional data can vary making the comprehensive HIE medical record potentially out of date. Second, aggregating data from multiple institutions creates administrative complexity with regard to HIPAA regulations. HIPAA requires each health care institution to maintain security of patient data. If an institution's data are "mixed" in the HIE database with data from other institutions, the responsibility of who ensures patient privacy and data security reverts to all HIE member institutions. HIPAA requirements make fulfilling health care organization obligations to insure patient privacy more difficult and complex. Third, when data are aggregated by a third party or HIE, the ability of the source institution to assert control over data contributed to the collective HIE is limited. If, for example, an institution desires to stop participating in an HIE because of concern for patient privacy and data security, it may be technically difficult and time consuming to selectively delete all data from one institution from the HIE database. The monolithic model is depicted in Figure 4.

The federated model is the most widely used design, allowing contributing institutions to maintain control over data for which they are responsible under HIPAA. In this model, institutional data resides only within each institution's system. The HIE database is small, containing only a master patient index (MPI) housing the identifiers for each patient in the form of each institution's unique patient record numbers along with only sufficient patient demographic data to facilitate accurate identification of individual patients with the same or similar names. This information is mapped to all of the institutional-specific patient identifiers in the exchange. Figure 5 depicts the federated model.

For example, a patient who has medical records at more than one institution in the HIE would have all their medical record numbers from the

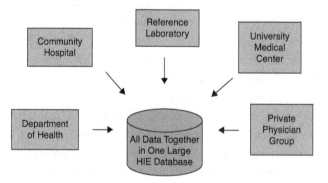

FIGURE 4 HIE Monolithic Model. Institutions periodically send copies of their clinical data to one central repository. Individual trans-institutional patient records are maintained in the central database where they can be accessed by authorized users.

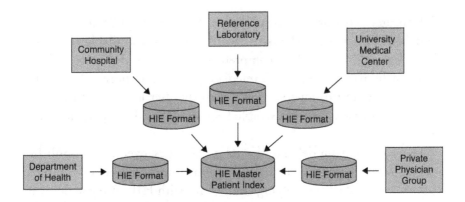

FIGURE 5 HIE Federated Model. Institutions maintain copies of their own data at their site in the format used by the health information exchange (HIE). Individual trans-institutional patient records are assembled in real time by searching all institutions' databases only when needed/requested by authorized users. Individual institutions can "op-out" of the HIE at any time by disabling access to their database.

various institutions where they have clinical data stored, linked together in the common MPI along with basic demographics such as address, date of birth, and social security number. This allows for fast and accurate identification of patients named "John Smith" because the MPI maintains only sufficient identifying information to ensure selection of the correct patient among all institutions in the exchange. "John Smith" would be identified from others with the same name by parameters such as date of birth, social security number. No clinical data are stored in the MPI. Clinical data are usually maintained in the proprietary format of the particular EHR system used by each institution. A copy of the same data is also maintained but is formatted in the standard used by all members of the HIE. For example, all HIE members could agree to code all laboratory test results using the LOINC standard described earlier. Each institution would create and maintain a database of all patients' laboratory results coded with LOINC. When a user requests a comprehensive record from the HIE, the system would query all of its institutional members in real time to send all the data available on a particular patient as identified using the MPI. In this way, when an HIE receives a records request on a particular patient, each institution sends data on the requested patient from the database where all clinical data are in the

HIE format. This process ensures that the data are collected securely, assembled into a comprehensive record, and made available to authorized users in real time. This comprehensive record is only accessible on a patient-by-patient basis for immediate patient care purposes; it is not copied to any institution's system. When the user logs out of the HIE, the comprehensive record assembled for that episode of patient care is deleted.

The federated model has several advantages over the monolithic model. With the federated model, each institution maintains complete control over its data, simplifying compliance with HIPAA regulations. If, for example, a data breach occurs in the database of an HIE that uses the monolithic model, responsibility for the data breach is not always clear. Data breaches in a federated system are always clearly attributable to a particular institution and not the HIE (unless there is a data breach of the MPI). Another benefit of the federated system is that trans-institutional data are up-to-the-minute accurate because each time a user requests access, the clinical data from all institutions are assembled in real time. Institutional HIT administrators typically favor the federated model. With this model, HIT administrators have the option of withdrawing from the HIE at any time in order to maintain control of their responsibilities for patient information and data security under HIPAA guidelines.

While communities with HIEs generally appreciate the benefits, the current reality is that most of the operating HIEs are heavily subsidized with federal research grant funding. The RHIOs that administer the HIEs and seek funding have not developed a business model that can be used in all communities in order to sustain their HIEs independent of federal funding. Some HIEs have developed services for payers, charging them for access to the comprehensive records available in the HIE. These services allow payers to increase their claims processing efficiency. Other HIEs have developed services to generate comprehensive quality reports to sell to payers desiring to track physician and health plan outcomes or to help them meet the meaningful use requirements for CMS financial eligibility incentives. Some communities are resistant to allowing payer access to a data resource they believe should be solely dedicated to improving patient care and quality.[61] An excellent example of this is the State of Vermont's 2006 law that prevented data miners from selling physicians' prescribing data to pharmaceutical companies who wanted the information to inform their marketing practices. In 2011, the law was struck down by the Supreme

Court on a First Amendment basis.[62] Physicians may feel uncomfortable participating in an exchange they know government, payers, or pharmaceutical companies may use for monitoring of individual practice outcomes and patterns. While the benefits of HIEs are documented and desirable, solving the cultural and business model issues will be essential to obtaining the national goal of a network of regional exchanges that will constitute the Nationwide Health Information Network.

The Veterans Administration Health Information System

No discussion of HIT, EHRs, and HIEs would be complete without noting the HIT system used by the Veterans Administration (VA). The VA is a model representing a single-payer health care system in the United States. For example, the VA HIT system supports only one payer, one pharmaceutical formulary, one provider group, and one supplier of laboratory testing. All VA physicians are employees of the same organization, so new policies and practices can be communicated, implemented, and monitored much more easily and efficiently than in U.S. multipayer, multiformulary, siloed system. Also, key is that the VA has one, universal EHR system with CPOE and CDSS. The VA EHR is able to code all data in one format that allows veterans who move from state to state to have their entire VA medical record seamlessly follow them. All these factors have allowed the VA to offer high-quality care at a relatively reasonable cost. Until the United States creates a single payer system and uses the same EHR universally, the larger system will suffer from the enormous complexity and costs of developing and maintaining multiple data standards to support the exchange of health information among institutions and across vendor platforms.

EHR Adoption Progress in the United States

One of the legislated functions of the ONC is to perform periodic surveys of EHR adoption. The ONC performs two national surveys. One surveys physician offices and the other surveys hospitals. The ONC defines two levels of adoption defined as "Basic" and "Full."[63] This distinction is

113

important because many other surveys report EHR adoption rates but do not define in any detail what "EHR adoption" means. The ONC survey uses an exacting definition of "Basic" and "Advanced" EHR adoption that produces results that are much more valid than surveys where "adoption" is not well defined. Figure 6 from the January 2012 ONC report to Congress, "Update on the Adoption of Health Information Technology and Related Efforts to Facilitate the Electronic Use and Exchange of Health Information," illustrates the rate of EHR "Basic" adoption among non-hospital-based physicians. These results demonstrate a steady increase in the adoption of "Basic" EHRs[64]:

> As of 2011, 34% of non-hospital-based physicians had adopted a "basic" EHR. This is double the adoption rate among non-hospital-based physicians in 2008. Adoption among primary care physicians, a key focus area of the HITECH Act, grew to approximately 40 percent; adoption among this same group has nearly doubled since 2008. These results are initial indications of the effects that the HITECH Act and CMS and ONC programs have had to date in accelerating the adoption of health IT and EHRs.[63]

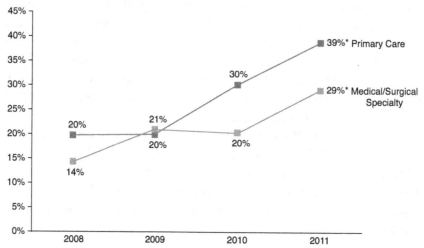

*Significantly higher than previous year estimate, or in the case of primary care all other physicians, at $p<0.05$. Adoption of "Basic" electronic health records as defined in: Hsiao CJ, et al. Electronic Medical Record/Electronic Health Record Systems of Non-hospital-based physicians: United States, 2009 and Preliminary 2010 State Estimates Health E Stats. National Center for Health Statistics, Centers for Disease Control.

FIGURE 6 Adoption of "Basic" Electronic Health Records Among Non-Hospital-Based Physicians.
Source: Reproduced from ONC report to Congress. Update on the Adoption of Health Information Technology and Related Efforts to Facilitate the Electronic Use and Exchange of Health Information: A Report to Congress. Jan 2012, Page 8.

Figure 7 from the ONC report noted above, illustrates the adoption rate of "Basic" EHRs among nonfederal acute care hospitals[64]:

The report states "Nearly 19 percent of non-federal acute care hospitals adopted a 'basic' EHR by 2010. This represents over a 50 percent increase in adoption among hospitals since 2008."[64]

The adoption rate of electronic prescribing or "e-prescribing" has been much more successful than the overall adoption of basic EHRs. The ONC report of 2012 further noted:

> Data from Surescripts, the nation's largest electronic prescribing network, shows that the percent of non-hospital based physicians active on the Surescripts network using an electronic health record has increased more than three-fold since 2008, to 44 percent. Pharmacies have reached near-universal adoption of electronic prescribing at 93 percent.[64]

The report also attributes much of the increase to the CMS financial incentive program for e-prescribing. Figures 8 and 9 from the January 2012 ONC report provide the adoption rates for e-prescribing by non-hospital-based physicians and retail community pharmacies.[64]

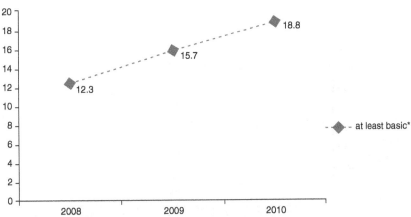

*Without physician notes and Nursing Assessments, as defined in Jha AK, et al. Use of Electronic Health Records in U.S. Hospitals. N Engl J Med. 2009 360;16.

FIGURE 7 Adoption of "Basic" Electronic Health Records Among Nonfederal Acute Care Hospitals.
Source: Reproduced from ONC report to Congress. Update on the Adoption of Health Information Technology and Related Efforts to Facilitate the Electronic Use and Exchange of Health Information: A Report to Congress. Jan 2012, Page 9.

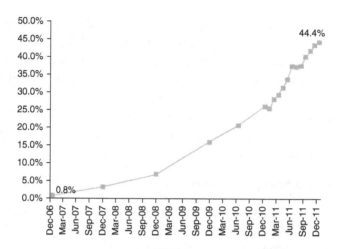

FIGURE 8 Adoption of Electronic Prescribing Through and Electronic Health Record Among Non-Hospital-Based Physicians.
Source: Reproduced from ONC report to Congress. Update on the Adoption of Health Information Technology and Related Efforts to Facilitate the Electronic Use and Exchange of Health Information: A Report to Congress. Jan 2012, Page 10.

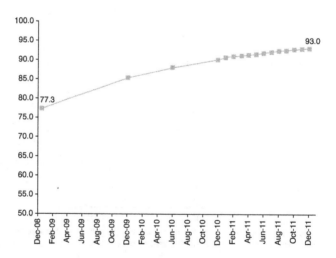

FIGURE 9 Adoption of Electronic Prescribing Among Retail Community Pharmacies.
Source: Reproduced from ONC report to Congress. Update on the Adoption of Health Information Technology and Related Efforts to Facilitate the Electronic Use and Exchange of Health Information: A Report to Congress. Jan 2012, Page 11.

Future Challenges

Although there is mounting evidence supporting the value of EHRs with CPOE and CDSS in several well-defined areas such as improving preventative care delivery, the extensive meta-analyses only report the combined average results. There have been several inconclusive and negative studies, and some that have actually shown patient harm associated with the installation of CPOE. In one of the most extensively reported, the mortality rate in a neonatal intensive care unit more than doubled after a CPOE system was installed at the University of Pittsburgh.[65] Much has been written about the reasons for this negative result and despite the finger pointing, there is virtually universal agreement that HIT can be very disruptive to work processes and work cultures resulting in significant harm to patients.[66] Some have called for more HIT standards and regulation to prevent these negative consequences in the same way as the U.S. Food and Drug Administration regulates medical devices.[67,68]

Due to the administrative and technical difficulties of achieving the Nationwide Health Information Network, proprietary entities have offered alternate approaches to develop "personal health records" (PHRs) through which patients create their own records in a standardized format. In these approaches, patients may physically carry records or make them available to caregivers via the Internet. Microsoft, Google, and many others have built such systems but with little marketing success. Google Health announced its shutdown on June 24, 2011, after only 3 years of operation. Google joins other lesser known firms that have decided to close down PHR services.[69] Design of existing PHRs requires patients to have a high level of health literacy and computer savvy. A major reason analysts believed Google Health failed was the newness of the concept for most people and the fact that PHRs are difficult to use and that many people find the necessary amount of data entry work necessary to complete their record to be too laborious.[70] One survey of patients found that only 7% had tried using a PHR and only about 3% continued to use them in 2011.[70] Other barriers to patient adoption include lack of personal health management tools (PHMT), the difficulty in achieving semantic interoperability such that PHMTs could be useful, problems vetting the identity of PHR users, patient privacy concerns, and perhaps most importantly, the lack of a business model to support the long-term operation of PHRs.[69]

In addition to physicians and patients affected by development and implementation of HIT, there are many other health care professionals and venues with significant complexities and characteristics that make HIT implementation challenging. Many of the same issues previously discussed in this chapter apply to these venues such as standardized data formats to facilitate data portability, work culture barriers, system expense, training issues, and other matters. For example, some emergency medical service (EMS) providers have begun to use a variety of portable EHRs to collect data at the scenes of patient incidents with systems designed to transmit data to receiving hospitals. The same issues that complicate the ease of universal HIE between health care institutions apply to the data exchange between EMS and hospital systems and will not be easily resolved.

To achieve the HIT goals of improving health care quality and reducing costs, extensive and rigorous work remains in the research and implementation arenas. After 50 years of efforts and most notably in the past 5 years, government, industry, and academia are only now recognizing the critically important and interdependent roles that standardization, administrative processes, and work cultures play in the HIT desired outcomes.

Key Terms for Review

Computerized Decision Support System (CDSS)

Computerized Physician Order Entry (CPOE)

Federated Model of Health Information Exchange

Health Information Exchange (HIE)

Health Information Technology for Economic and Clinical Health Act (HITECH Act)

Meaningful Use

Monolithic Model of Health Information Exchange

Office of The National Coordinator for Health Information Technology (ONC)

Regional Health Information Organization (RHIO)

References

1. Bush GW. Executive Order: Incentives for the Use of Health Information Technology and Establishing the Position of the National Health Information Technology Coordinator. 2004; http://georgewbush-whitehouse.archives.gov/news/releases/2004/04/20040427-4.html. Accessed September 25, 2012.

2. One Hundred Eleventh Congress of the United States of America. *The American Recovery and Reinvestment Act.* Washington, DC; U.S. Government Printing Office; 2009.

3. The Life Sciences Panel of the President's Science Advisory Committee. *Some New Technologies and their Promise for the Life Sciences.* Washington, DC: The White House; January 23, 1963.

4. Duke Evidence-based Practice Center. *Enabling Health Care Decisionmaking through Clinical Decision Support and Knowledge Management.* Rockville, MD: Agency for Healthcare Research and Quality, U.S. Department of Health and Human Services; 2012.

5. McDonald CJ. Protocol-based computer reminders, the quality of care and the non-perfectability of man. *N Engl J Med.* 1976;295(24):1351–1355.

6. Yount RJ, Vries JK, Councill CD. The Medical Archival System: an Information Retrieval System Based on Distributed Parallel Processing. *Info Proces Management.* 1991;27(4):1–11.

7. Gardner RM, Pryor TA, Warner HR. The HELP hospital information system: update 1998. *Int J Med Inform.* 1999;54(3):169–182.

8. Pryor TA, Gardner RM, Clayton PD, Warner HR. The HELP system. *J Med Syst.* 1983;7(2):87–102.

9. Higgins SB, Jiang K, Swindell BB, Bernard GR. A graphical ICU workstation. *Proc Annu Symp Comput Appl Med Care.* 1991; 783–787.

10. Giuse DA, Mickish A. Increasing the availability of the computerized patient record. *Proc AMIA Annu Fall Symp.* 1996; 633–637.

11. Stead WW, Hammond WE. Computer-based medical records: the centerpiece of TMR. *MD Comput.* 1988;5(5):48–62.

12. Greenes RA, Pappalardo AN, Marble CW, Barnett GO. Design and implementation of a clinical data management system. *Comput Biomed Res.* 1969;2(5):469–485.

13. United States Department of Health and Human Services. Certified Health IT Product List. 2012; http://oncchpl.force.com/ehrcert?q=CHPL. Accessed September 28, 2012.

14. HITECH Programs and Advisory Committees. Health IT Adoption Programs. http://www.healthit.gov/policy-researchers-implementers/health-it-adoption-programs. Accessed January 20, 2012.

15. Campbell EM, Guappone KP, Sittig DF, Dykstra RH, Ash JS. Computerized provider order entry adoption: implications for clinical workflow. *J Gen Intern Med.* 2009;24(1):21–26.

16. Bloomrosen M, Starren J, Lorenzi NM, Ash JS, Patel VL, Shortliffe EH. Anticipating and addressing the unintended consequences of health IT and policy: a report from the AMIA 2009 Health Policy Meeting. *J Am Med Inform Assoc.* 2011;18(1):82–90.

17. Ash JS, Stavri PZ, Dykstra R, Fournier L. Implementing computerized physician order entry: the importance of special people. *Int J Med Inform.* 2003;69(2–3):235–250.

18. Chaudhry B, Wang J, Wu S, et al. Systematic review: impact of health information technology on quality, efficiency, and costs of medical care. *Ann Intern Med.* 2006;144(10):742–752.

19. Ash JS, Bates DW. Factors and forces affecting EHR system adoption: report of a 2004 ACMI discussion. *J Am Med Inform Assoc.* 2005;12(1):8–12.

20. Connolly C. Cedars-Sinai Doctors Clinic to Pen and Paper. *The Washington Post.* March 21, 2005:A01. Available from http://gunston.gmu.edu/health-science/740/Presentations/cedars-sinai%20cpoe%20washpost%203-21-05.pdf. Accessed April 21, 2013.

21. Dexter PR, Perkins S, Overhage JM, Maharry K, Kohler RB, McDonald CJ. A computerized reminder system to increase the use of preventive care for hospitalized patients. *N Engl J Med.* 2001;345(13):965–970.

22. Weiner M, Callahan CM, Tierney WM, et al. Using information technology to improve the health care of older adults. *Ann Intern Med.* 2003;139(5 Pt 2): 430–436.

23. Dexter PR, Perkins SM, Maharry KS, Jones K, McDonald CJ. Inpatient computer-based standing orders vs physician reminders to increase influenza and pneumococcal vaccination rates: a randomized trial. *JAMA.* 2004;292(19):2366–2371.

24. Overhage JM, Dexter PR, Perkins SM, et al. A randomized, controlled trial of clinical information shared from another institution. *Ann Emerg Med.* 2002;39(1):14–23.

25. One Hundred Eleventh Congress of the United States of America. Health Information Technology for Economic and Clinical Health Act. 2009; http://www.hhs.gov/ocr/privacy/hipaa/understanding/coveredentities/hitechact.pdf. Accessed September 25, 2012.

26. The Office of the National Coordinator for Health Information Technology (ONC). About ONC. 2012; http://healthit.hhs.gov/portal/server.pt/community/healthit_hhs_gov_onc/1200. Accessed November 24, 2012.

27. The Office of the National Coordinator for Health Information Technology (ONC). ONC Organizational Structure. 2012; http://healthit.hhs.gov/portal/server.pt/community/healthit_hhs_gov__organization/1512. Accessed November 24, 2012.

28. United States Department of Health and Human Services. HITECH Programs & Advisory Committees. http://www.healthit.gov/policy-researchers-implementers/federal-advisory-committees-facas. Accessed September 24, 2012.

29. Centers for Medicare and Medicaid Services. Eligible Hospital Information. 2012; http://www.cms.gov/Regulations-and-Guidance/Legislation/EHRIncentivePrograms/Eligible_Hospital_Information.html. Accessed October 30, 2012.

30. Centers for Medicare and Medicaid Services. EHR Incentive Program for Medicare Hospitals. 2012; http://www.cms.gov/Outreach-and-Education/Medicare-Learning-Network-MLN/MLNProducts/downloads/EHR_TipSheet_Medicare_Hosp.pdf. Accessed October 30, 2012.

31. Centers for Medicare and Medicaid Services. Medicaid Hospital Incentive Payments Calculations. 2012; http://www.cms.gov/Outreach-and-Education/Medicare-Learning-Network-MLN/MLNProducts/downloads/Medicaid_Hosp_Incentive_Payments_Tip_Sheets.pdf. Accessed October 30, 2012.

32. Centers for Medicare and Medicaid Services. Flow Chart to Help Eligible Professionals (EP) Determine Eligibility for the Medicare and Medicaid Electronic Health Record (EHR) Incentive Programs. 2012; https://www.cms.gov/Regulations-and-Guidance/Legislation/EHRIncentivePrograms/downloads/eligibility_flow_chart.pdf. Accessed December 21, 2012.

33. Centers for Medicare and Medicaid Services. EHR Incentive Programs. 2012; http://www.cms.gov/Regulations-and-Guidance/Legislation/EHRIncentivePrograms/index.html?redirect=/ehrincentiveprograms/. Accessed September 24, 2012.

34. Centers for Medicare and Medicaid Services. Medicare Electronic Health Record Incentive Program for Eligible Professionals. 2012; http://www.cms.gov/Outreach-and-Education/Medicare-Learning-Network-MLN/MLNProducts/Downloads/CMS_eHR_Tip_Sheet.pdf. Accessed December 22, 2012.

35. Centers for Medicare and Medicaid Services. An Introduction to the Medicaid EHR Incentive Program for Eligible Professionals. 2012; http://www.cms.gov/Regulations-and-Guidance/Legislation/EHRIncentivePrograms/Downloads/EHR_Medicaid_Guide_Remediated_2012.pdf. Accessed December 22, 2012.

36. Centers for Medicare and Medicaid Services. An Introduction to the Medicare EHR Incentive Program for Eligible Professionals. 2012; http://www.cms.gov/Regulations-and-Guidance/Legislation/EHRIncentivePrograms/Downloads/Beginners_Guide.pdf. Accessed December 22, 2012.

37. Centers for Medicare and Medicaid Services. Medicaid Electronic Health Record Incentive Payments for Eligible Professionals. 2012; http://www.cms.gov/Outreach-and-Education/Medicare-Learning-Network-MLN/MLNProducts/Downloads/EHRIP_Eligible_Professionals_Tip_Sheet.pdf. Accessed December 22, 2012.

38. Centers for Medicare and Medicaid Services. Meaningful Use. 2012; http://www.cms.gov/Regulations-and-Guidance/Legislation/EHRIncentivePrograms/Meaningful_Use.html. Accessed September 24, 2012.

39. Centers for Medicare and Medicaid Services. Medicare and Medicaid EHR Incentive Program Basics. 2012; http://www.cms.gov/Regulations-and-Guidance/Legislation/EHRIncentivePrograms/Basics.html. Accessed October 30, 2012.

40. United States Department of Health and Human Services. Meaningful Use. 2012; http://www.healthit.gov/policy-researchers-implementers/meaningful-use. Accessed December 21, 2012.

41. Centers for Medicare and Medicaid Services. Eligible Professional Meaningful Use Table of Contents Core and Menu Set Objectives. 2012; https://www.cms.gov/Regulations-and-Guidance/Legislation/EHRIncentivePrograms/downloads/EP-MU-TOC.pdf. Accessed October 30, 2012.

42. Centers for Medicare and Medicaid Services. Eligible Hospital and CAH Meaningful Use Table of Contents Core and Menu Set Objectives. 2012; http://www.cms.gov/Regulations-and-Guidance/Legislation/EHRIncentivePrograms/downloads/Hosp_CAH_MU-TOC.pdf. Accessed October 30, 2012.

43. United States Department of Health and Human Services. Stage 1 vs. Stage 2 Comparison Table for Eligible Professionals. 2012; http://www.cms.gov/Regulations-and-Guidance/Legislation/EHRIncentivePrograms/Downloads/Stage1vsStage2CompTablesforEP.pdf. Accessed September 24, 2012.

44. United States Department of Health and Human Services. Stage 1 vs. Stage 2 Comparison Table for Eligible Hospitals and CAHs. 2012; http://www.cms.gov/Regulations-and-Guidance/Legislation/EHRIncentivePrograms/Downloads/Stage1vsStage2CompTablesforHospitals.pdf. Accessed September 25, 2012.

45. Dukette D, Cornish D. *The Essential 20: Twenty Components of an Excellent Health Care Team.* Pittsburgh, PA: RoseDog Books; 2009: 72–74.

46. Parthasarathy S. Sleep and the medical profession. *Curr Opin Pulm Med.* 2005;11(6):507–512.

47. Institute of Medicine. *Free Executive Summary: Beyond Expert-Based Practice. IOM Annual Meeting Summary: Evidence-Based Medicine and the Changing Nature of Healthcare.* Washington, DC: The National Academies Press; 2008: 18–19.

48. Friedman CP. What informatics is and isn't. *J Am Med Inform Assoc.* 2012;0:1–3.

49. Evans RS, Pestotnik SL, Classen DC, et al. A computer-assisted management program for antibiotics and other antiinfective agents. *N Engl J Med.* 1998;338(4):232–238.

50. Tierney WM, Dexter PR, Gramelspacher GP, Perkins AJ, Zhou XH, Wolinsky FD. The effect of discussions about advance directives on patients' satisfaction with primary care. *J Gen Intern Med.* 2001;16(1):32–40.

51. Gardner RM. Computerized clinical decision-support in respiratory care. *Respir Care.* 2004;49(4):378–386; discussion 386–378.

52. Tierney WM, Miller ME, Overhage JM, McDonald CJ. Physician inpatient order writing on microcomputer workstations. Effects on resource utilization. *JAMA.* 1993;269(3):379–383.

53. Kho AN, Dexter P, Lemmon L, et al. Connecting the dots: creation of an electronic regional infection control network. *Stud Health Technol Inform.* 2007;129(Pt 1):213–217.

54. Kho A, Dexter P, Warvel J, Commiskey M, Wilson S, McDonald CJ. Computerized reminders to improve isolation rates of patients with drug-resistant infections: design and preliminary results. *AMIA Annu Symp Proc.* 2005; 390–394.

55. Rosenman M, Wang J, Dexter P, Overhage JM. Computerized reminders for syphilis screening in an urban emergency department. *AMIA Annu Symp Proc.* 2003; 987.

56. Kroth PJ, Dexter PR, Overhage JM, et al. A computerized decision support system improves the accuracy of temperature capture from nursing personnel at the bedside. *AMIA Annu Symp Proc.* 2006; 444–448.

57. Agency for Healthcare Research and Quality. Evidence Report/Tecghnology Assessment Number 203: Enabling Health Care Decisionmaking Through Clinical Decision Support and Knowledge. 2012; http://www.ahrq.gov/clinic/tp/knowmgttp.htm. Accessed October 29, 2012.

58. Markle Foundation. The Common Framework: Technical Issues and Requirements for Implementation. 2006; http://www.markle.org/sites/default/files/T1_TechIssues.pdf. Accessed December 21, 2012.

59. Lin MC, Vreeman DJ, McDonald CJ, Huff SM. Auditing consistency and usefulness of LOINC use among three large institutions - using version spaces for grouping LOINC codes. *J Biomed Inform.* 2012;45(4):658–666.

60. National Library of Medicine. UMLS Quick Start Guide. 2012; http://www.nlm.nih.gov/research/umls/quickstart.html. Accessed January 11, 2013.

61. Sorrell WH. Supreme Court Strikes Down Vermont Prescription Privacy Law. 2011; http://www.atg.state.vt.us/news/supreme-court-strikes-down-vermont-prescription-privacy-law.php. Accessed November 24, 2012.

62. The Supreme Court of the United States. Sorrell, Attorney General of Vermont, et al. vs. IMS Health Inc. et al. 2011; http://www.supremecourt.gov/opinions/10pdf/10-779.pdf. Accessed January 12, 2013.

63. Hsiao CJ, Hing E, Socey TC, Cai B. Electronic health record systems and intent to apply for meaningful use incentives among office-based physician practices: United States, 2001–2011. *NCHS Data Brief.* 2011;79:1–8. Available from http://www.cdc.gov/nchs/data/databriefs/db79.htm. Accessed April 19, 2013.

64. The Office of the National Coordinator for Health Information Technology (ONC). Update on the Adoption of Health Information Technology and Related Efforts to Facilitate the Electronic Use and Exchange of Health Information: A Report to Congress. January 2012; http://healthit.hhs.gov/portal/server.pt/gateway/PTARGS_0_0_4383_1239_15610_43/http%3B/wci-pubcontent/publish/onc/public_communities/p_t/resources_and_public_affairs/reports/reports_portlet/files/january2012__update_on_hit_adoption_report_to_congress.pdf. Accessed September 29, 2012.

65. Han YY, Carcillo JA, Venkataraman ST, et al. Unexpected increased mortality after implementation of a commercially sold computerized physician order entry system. *Pediatrics.* 2005;116(6):1506–1512.

66. Sittig DF, Ash JS, Zhang J, Osheroff JA, Shabot MM. Lessons from "Unexpected increased mortality after implementation of a commercially sold computerized physician order entry system." *Pediatrics.* 2006;118(2): 797–801.

67. Miller RA, Gardner RM. Summary recommendations for responsible monitoring and regulation of clinical software systems. American Medical Informatics Association, The Computer-based Patient Record Institute, The

Medical Library Association, The Association of Academic Health Science Libraries, The American Health Information Management Association, and The American Nurses Association. *Ann Intern Med.* 1997;127(9):842–845.

68. Miller RA, Gardner RM. Recommendations for responsible monitoring and regulation of clinical software systems. American Medical Informatics Association, Computer-based Patient Record Institute, Medical Library Association, Association of Academic Health Science Libraries, American Health Information Management Association, American Nurses Association. *J Am Med Inform Assoc.* 1997;4(6):442–457.

69. Rishel W, Booz RH. Google Health Shutdown Underscores Uncertain Future of PHRs. 2011; http://www.gartner.com/resources/214600/214682/google_health_shutdown_under_214682.pdf. Accessed October 29, 2012.

70. Lohr S. Google Is Closing Its Health Records Service. *The New York Times.* June 24, 2011.

HIPAA and HITECH

LEARNING OBJECTIVES

After completing class sessions based on this chapter, a student will:

- Understand the detailed requirements of the Privacy and Security Rules under the Health Insurance Portability and Accountability Act of 1996 (HIPAA), and the differences between the two rules.
- Know what a covered entity and a business associate are and how they relate to each other.
- Recognize what types of use and disclosure of protected health information (PHI) are permitted and prohibited by HIPAA.
- Be familiar with individuals' rights to their own PHI.
- Learn about the Breach Notification Rule and how it applies to healthcare organizations.
- Be acquainted with the safeguards, standards, and specifications of the Security Rule and how they relate to each other.
- Discover the civil and criminal penalties that may result from HIPAA violations.

INTRODUCTION

It is a national strategic goal to promote the adoption and use of electronic medical records (EMRs) throughout the healthcare system. The Centers for Medicare and Medicaid Services (CMS) has embarked upon a multiyear program of financial incentives to encourage the "meaningful use" of EMRs by hospitals and physicians. The United States is slowly moving toward the universal deployment of EMRs, computerized physician order entry (CPOE), health information exchanges (HIEs), and other forms of health information technology already achieved in other developed countries.

New technologies are constantly emerging. The healthcare industry is relying more and more on electronic information systems to pay claims, answer eligibility questions, provide health information, and conduct a host of other administrative and clinically based functions. This means that healthcare workers can be more mobile and efficient, while patients can be better informed and more involved in their own health care. This widespread dispersal of sensitive, personal healthcare information among multiple organizations, facilities, and personnel presents serious risks to security and privacy.

The HIPAA of 1996 was enacted to protect against these threats. The scope of HIPAA was modestly expanded by provisions of the Health Information Technology for Economic and Clinical Health (HITECH) Act, passed into law in 2009.

Under HIPAA's authority, the Department of Health and Human Services (DHHS) issued regulations that established national Standards for Privacy of Individually Identifiable Health Information (the Privacy Rule) and Security Standards for the Protection of Electronic Protected Health Information (the Security Rule).

WHO IS COVERED BY HIPAA

The Privacy and Security Rules apply to what are called "covered entities" and to the "business associates" of those entities. Covered entities encompass three categories of organizations and individuals.

Healthcare Providers

Every healthcare provider, regardless of size, that electronically transmits health information in connection with certain transactions, is a covered entity. These transactions include claims, benefit eligibility inquiries, referral authorization requests, or other transactions for which DHHS has established standards under the HIPAA Transactions Rule. Using electronic technology, such as email, does not mean a healthcare provider is a covered entity; the transmission must be in connection with a standard transaction.

The Privacy Rule covers a healthcare provider whether it electronically transmits these transactions directly or uses a billing service or other third party to do so on its behalf. Healthcare providers include all "providers of services" (e.g., institutional providers such as hospitals) and "providers of medical or health services" (e.g., noninstitutional providers such as physicians, dentists, and other practitioners) as defined by Medicare, and any other person or organization that furnishes, bills, or is paid for health care.

Health Plans

Individual and group plans that provide or pay the cost of medical care are covered entities. This includes health, dental, vision, and prescription drug insurers; health maintenance organizations (HMOs); Medicare, Medicaid, and Medicare Advantage and Medicare supplement insurers; and long-term care insurers. Health plans also include employer-sponsored group health plans, government and church-sponsored health plans, and multi-employer health plans.

Healthcare Clearinghouses

The healthcare system relies on organizations that process health information received from a client in a nonstandard format into a standard format, or from a standard format into a nonstandard format. The entities that perform these services are billing services, repricing companies, community health management information systems, and value-added networks and switches. Their clients typically are health plans and healthcare providers.

All these entities must comply with the Rules to protect the privacy and security of health information and provide individuals with certain rights with respect to their health information. If an entity is not a covered entity, it does not have to comply with the Privacy Rule or the Security Rule.

The term "business associate" applies to a person or organization (other than a covered entity's own employees) who does work or provides services for a covered entity that involves the use or disclosure of individually identifiable health information. Examples of business associate services are claims processing, data analysis, utilization review, and billing. Persons or organizations are not considered business associates if their functions or services do not involve the use or disclosure of PHI, and where any access to PHI by such persons would be incidental, if at all.

When a covered entity uses an independent contractor or other non-employee to perform "business associate" services or activities, the Rules require that the entity enter into a formal contract with the associate that includes specific information safeguards. The contract may not authorize the business associate to make any use or disclosure of PHI that would violate the Rules.

A covered entity violates the Security Rule if it knows of a pattern of activity or practice of its business associate that constitutes a material breach or violation of the business associate's obligations under the business associate contract, unless the covered entity takes reasonable steps to cure the breach or end the violation. If such steps are unsuccessful, the covered entity must terminate the contract.

The HIPAA Privacy and Security rules, as well as the civil monetary and criminal penalties, apply directly to business associates. These obligations and risks make it essential that covered entities and their business associates enter into a close dialogue with each other about their compliance efforts. It would be very easy for the inadvertent actions of one to create serious legal liabilities for the other.

HIPAA PRIVACY RULE

The purpose of the Privacy Rule is to ensure that the personal health information of individuals, referred to as PHI, is properly protected, while still allowing the flow of health information that is vital to the delivery of quality health care and the protection of the public's well-being. The Rule aims to strike a balance between the essential systemic uses of that information and the privacy of the people served by the healthcare system.

The Privacy Rule standards address the use and disclosure of PHI by covered entities, as well as the rights of patients to understand and control how their health information is used. Within the DHHS, the responsibility for implementing and enforcing the Privacy Rule has been delegated to the Office for Civil Rights (OCR).

WHAT INFORMATION IS PROTECTED BY THE PRIVACY RULE

The Privacy Rule protects all "individually identifiable health information" held or transmitted by a covered entity or its business associate, in any form or media, whether electronic, paper, or oral. The Privacy Rule calls this information PHI. This is information that concerns an individual's past, present, or future physical or mental health or condition; the provision of healthcare services to the individual; and the past, present, or future payment for those services—and that identifies the individual. Typical identification data points are name, address, birth date, and Social Security number.

There are no restrictions on the use or disclosure of de-identified information—information that neither identifies nor provides a reasonable basis for identifying an individual.

WHAT THE PRIVACY RULE PROHIBITS

The fundamental purpose of the Privacy Rule is to define and limit the circumstances in which an individual's PHI may be used or disclosed by a covered entity or its business associates. A covered entity may use or disclose PHI only when the Privacy Rule requires or permits it, or when the affected individual has given his or her written authorization.

REQUIRED DISCLOSURE OF PHI

There are only two situations in which a covered entity must disclose PHI. The first is when the affected individual specifically requests access to or disclosure of his or her PHI. The second is when the DHHS seeks access in the course of a compliance investigation or review, or an enforcement action.

PERMITTED DISCLOSURE OF PHI

There are six situations in which a covered entity may, but is not required to, use or disclose PHI without the affected individual's authorization.

1. When it discloses PHI to the individual who is the subject of the information.
2. For use in the entity's own treatment, payment, and healthcare operations activities.

    Treatment is the provision, coordination, or management of health care and related services for an individual by one or more healthcare providers, including consultation between providers regarding a patient and referral of a patient by one provider to another.

    Payment encompasses activities of a health plan to obtain premiums, determine or fulfill responsibilities for coverage and provision of benefits, and furnish or obtain reimbursement for healthcare delivered to an individual as well as activities of a healthcare provider to obtain payment or be reimbursed for the provision of health care to an individual.

    Healthcare operations are any of the following activities: (a) quality assessment and improvement activities, including case management and care coordination; (b) competency assurance activities, including provider or health plan performance evaluation, credentialing, and accreditation; (c) conducting or arranging for medical reviews, audits, or legal services, including fraud and abuse detection and compliance programs; (d) specified insurance functions, such as underwriting, risk rating, and reinsuring risk; (e) business planning, development, management, and administration; and (f) business management and general administrative activities of the entity, including but not limited to, de-identifying PHI, creating a limited data set, and certain fundraising for the benefit of the covered entity.

3. When the affected individual has the opportunity to agree with or object to the disclosure.

   Informal permission may be obtained by asking the individual outright, or by circumstances that clearly give the individual the opportunity to agree, acquiesce, or object. Where the individual is incapacitated, in an emergency situation, or not available, covered entities generally may make such uses and disclosures if, in the exercise of their professional judgment, the use or disclosure is determined to be in the best interests of the individual.

4. When the use or disclosure is incidental to an otherwise permitted use or disclosure, the entity has reasonable privacy safeguards in place, and the disclosed information is the "minimum necessary."

5. When the use or disclosure is on the list of "national priority purposes." These include legally required (by statute, regulation, or court order) public health activities; situations involving victims of abuse, neglect, or domestic violence; health oversight activities (audits and investigations); judicial and administrative proceedings; certain law enforcement purposes; decedents; organ donations; research; serious threats to individual or public health and safety; essential government functions; and workers' compensation.

6. When it is in the form of a "limited data set" from which specified direct identifiers of individuals and their relatives, household members, and employers have been removed.

AUTHORIZATION ALLOWING USE OR DISCLOSURE

If the Privacy Rule does not require or permit use or disclosure of PHI, the authorization of the affected individual must be obtained. An authorization must be written in plain language, and contain specific information regarding the PHI to be disclosed or used, the persons who will disclose or use the PHI, the expiration date of the authorization, and the individual's right to revoke it in writing, among other terms. The authorization may extend to the covered entity or one of its agents. Typically, an authorization would be necessary for disclosures to a life insurer for coverage purposes, disclosures to an employer of the results of a pre-employment physical or lab test, or disclosures to a pharmaceutical firm for their own marketing purposes.

BASIC "MINIMUM NECESSARY" PRINCIPLE OF THE PRIVACY RULE

The Privacy Rule applies a single basic principle to the use and disclosure of PHI, whether it is required, permitted, or authorized: the covered entity must make reasonable efforts to use, disclose, and request only the minimum amount of PHI needed to accomplish its intended purpose. The entity must develop and implement policies and procedures to reasonably limit the uses and disclosures to the *minimum necessary*. These are some examples.

- Access and usage should be limited on the basis of the specific roles of each employee. Policies and procedures should identify the persons, or classes of persons, in the workforce who need access to PHI to perform their duties, the categories of PHI to which access is needed, and any conditions under which that access should be allowed.
- There should be formal limits on access allowed through routine, recurring disclosures, or requests for disclosures. In these circumstances, individual review of each disclosure would not be necessary.
- A covered entity may assume that a PHI request is for the "minimum necessary" when it comes from another covered entity, a public official, a professional (lawyer, accountant) who is a business associate of the covered entity, or an authenticated researcher.

NOTICE OF PRIVACY PRACTICES

Each covered entity, with certain exceptions, must provide a notice of its privacy practices. The notice must contain several elements: a description of the ways in which the entity may use or disclose the PHI, the entity's duties to protect privacy, the privacy rights of individuals, and a contact for seeking more information and making complaints. The Privacy Rule specifies how a covered entity must distribute this notice to direct treatment providers, other healthcare providers, and health plans. This is a sample Notice of Privacy Practices offered by the American Medical Association: http://www.ama-assn.org/resources/doc/hipaa/privacy-practices.doc.

INDIVIDUALS' RIGHTS TO THEIR PHI

Individuals have rights with regard to their PHI.

With a few exceptions, individuals have the right to review and obtain a copy of their PHI. They have the right to request that a covered entity amend their PHI when they believe it to be inaccurate or incomplete. If the request is denied, covered entities must put the denial in writing and allow the individual to submit a statement of disagreement for inclusion in the record. Individuals have a right to an accounting of the disclosures of their PHI by a covered entity or its business associates.

Individuals have the right to request that a covered entity restrict its use or disclosure of PHI to the following: for treatment, payment, or healthcare operations; to persons involved in the individual's health care or payment for health care; or to family members or others entitled to information about the individual's general condition, location, or death. A covered entity is under no obligation to agree to requests for restrictions.

Individuals have the right to request that they receive communications of PHI by different means than those normally used by the covered entity. For instance, an individual may request that a provider communicate with the individual at a designated address or phone number.

COVERED ENTITIES' IMPLEMENTATION OF THE PRIVACY RULE

Every covered entity must take concrete measures to satisfy the requirements of the Privacy Rule. The scope and detail of those measures will vary according to the nature of the entity's business and its size and resources. The most fundamental step is the development and implementation of appropriate privacy policies and procedures. The covered entity must designate a privacy official to be responsible for overseeing the policies and procedures, for disseminating privacy information, and for receiving complaints.

A covered entity must train all its employees on the privacy policies and procedures that bear on the performance of their job functions. It also must institute and apply appropriate sanctions against employees who violate its privacy policies and procedures or the Privacy Rule.

A covered entity must mitigate, to the extent practicable, the harmful effects that may have been caused by the use or disclosure of PHI by its employees or business associates in violation of its privacy policies and procedures or the Privacy Rule.

A covered entity must maintain reasonable and appropriate administrative, technical, and physical safeguards to prevent intentional or unintentional use or disclosure of PHI in violation of the Privacy Rule. The Security Rule provides greater detail about these safeguards.

A covered entity must have in place procedures for individuals to complain about its compliance with its privacy policies and procedures and with the Privacy Rule. It must explain those procedures in its privacy practices notice, and identify the person to whom individuals can submit their complaints.

A covered entity may not retaliate against a person for exercising rights provided by the Privacy Rule, or for opposing an act or practice that the person believes in good faith violates the Privacy Rule.

A covered entity must maintain, for 6 years after the date of their creation or their last effective date, whichever is later, its privacy policies and procedures, its privacy practices notices, the disposition of complaints, and other actions, activities, and designations that the Privacy Rule requires to be documented.

BREACH NOTIFICATION

In 2009, the HITECH Act added what is called the Breach Notification Rule. This rule requires that covered entities and their business associates provide notification following a breach of unsecured PHI. Similar breach notification provisions are implemented and enforced by the Federal Trade Commission against vendors of personal health records and their third-party service providers.

A breach is defined as an impermissible use or disclosure under the Privacy Rule that compromises the security or privacy of the PHI to the extent that it poses a significant risk of financial, reputational, or other harm to the affected individual. There are three exceptions to the definition of "breach."

1. The unintentional acquisition, access, or use of PHI by an employee of a covered entity or business associate.
2. The inadvertent disclosure of PHI from a person authorized to access PHI at a covered entity or business associate to another person authorized to access PHI at the covered entity or business associate.
3. A covered entity or business associate has a good faith belief that the unauthorized individual, to whom the impermissible disclosure was made, would not have been able to retain the information.

Covered entities and business associates need only provide notification if the breach involved unsecured PHI. Unsecured PHI is health information that has not been rendered unusable, unreadable, or indecipherable to unauthorized individuals through the use of a technology or methodology such as encryption or destruction.

Following a breach of unsecured PHI, covered entities must provide notification of the breach to affected individuals, the DHHS, and, in certain circumstances, to the media. In addition, business associates must notify covered entities when a breach has occurred.

Individual notice. Covered entities must notify affected individuals within 60 days following the discovery of a breach of unsecured PHI. Covered entities must provide this individual notice in written form by first-class mail, or alternatively, by email if the affected individual has agreed to receive such notices electronically. If the covered entity has insufficient or out-of-date contact information for 10 or more individuals, the covered entity must provide substitute individual notice by either posting the notice on the home page of its website or by providing the notice in major print or broadcast media where the affected individuals likely reside.

Media notice. Covered entities that experience a breach affecting more than 500 residents of a single state are, in addition to notifying the affected individuals, required to provide notice to prominent media outlets serving the state.

DHHS notice. In addition to notifying affected individuals and the media, covered entities must notify the DHHS of breaches of unsecured PHI. They will do this by visiting the DHHS website and electronically submitting a breach report form. To see how this can be done, visit this location: http://ocrnotifications.hhs.gov/.

To review the steps in deciding whether a breach notification is necessary as the following questions:

1. Was the incident a breach?
2. Did the incident fit one of the three exceptions to the definition of a breach?
3. Does the breach require notification?
4. Was the breach unauthorized?
5. Was the PHI that was accessed or disclosed unsecure?
6. Has the breach resulted in financial, reputational, or other harm to the affected individual?

Then, the affected individual must be notified.

These are examples of breaches that would require notification:

- Fax with unsecure PHI sent to the wrong number
- Lost laptop with unsecure PHI
- Lost flash drive with unsecure PHI

- Email with unsecure PHI sent to wrong address
- Intentional access to more PHI than permitted under HIPAA exception
- Access to personal medical record without good reason
- Sharing PHI with persons outside the organization who have no need to see it
- Sending PHI to an outside entity with no business associate agreement

HIPAA SECURITY RULE

The Security Rule is the other half of HIPAA. It applies to the same organizations as the Privacy Rule: covered entities, business associates, and subcontractors. However, this rule deals only with the security of electronic protected health information (E-PHI). This is in contrast with the Privacy Rule, which applies to all forms of PHI—electronic, written, or oral. The Security Rule does not apply to PHI transmitted orally or in writing.

Most healthcare organizations manage and transmit large volumes of electronic information other than E-PHI (e.g., financial, personnel, non-clinical operations). They are not required to implement the provisions of the Security Rule with regard to those kinds of information. However, many organizations find it easier to put the Rule into practice throughout their electronic systems, covering all forms of electronic information.

The requirements of the Security Rule are rationally organized. There are three broad categories of "safeguards"—administrative, physical, and technical. Within each category, there are "standards" that must be followed. For most of the standards, there are one or more "specifications" that offer more detail on how to implement the standard. Where there is no specification, the standard itself is deemed to provide enough guidance on implementation. Most of the specifications are "required"; a few are designated "addressable." The addressable specifications may be implemented as written or through closely restricted alternative means.

Due to the nature of computer systems, both hardware and software, security can be achieved through a variety of means. It is impossible to prescribe a single universal approach that all healthcare organizations could use. Accordingly, the HIPAA regulations allow some flexibility to those organizations in carrying out the Security Rule requirements. In deciding how much leeway they have, the organizations may take into account:

- The size, complexity, and capabilities of the organization
- Its technical infrastructure, hardware, and software security capabilities

- The costs to the organization of possible security measures
- The probability and criticality of potential risks to E-PHI

In addition, when they are making decisions about exactly how they will implement security measures, covered entities should keep in mind the end goals of the Security Rule.

- Ensure the confidentiality, integrity, and availability of all E-PHI that the covered entity creates, receives, maintains, or transmits.
- Protect against any reasonably anticipated threats or hazards to the security or integrity of the entity's E-PHI.
- Protect against any reasonably anticipated uses or disclosures of such information that are not permitted or required under the Privacy Rule.
- Ensure compliance with the Security Rule by the covered entity's employees.

SAFEGUARDS, STANDARDS, AND SPECIFICATIONS

The DHHS recommends that covered entities carry out a risk analysis to determine which security measures are reasonable and appropriate for their particular organization. In addition, they should conduct ongoing reviews to track access to E-PHI, recognize security incidents, evaluate the effectiveness of existing security measures, and reassess potential risks to E-PHI security. A good risk analysis procedure includes:

- Identifying the areas of highest risk to E-PHI security.
- Evaluating the likelihood and impact of those risks.
- Implementing appropriate security measures to address the risks identified.
- Documenting the chosen security measures and the rationale for adopting them.

With a better understanding of where its greatest security risks lie, a covered entity can proceed to develop and implement standards and specifications designed to address them.

In the modern world of healthcare delivery and financing, the protection of information privacy and security inevitably involves highly sophisticated technology systems. To be able to competently implement the following standards, it is important to have a good understanding of how those systems function. A Compliance Officer responsible for ensuring an organization's conformity with a wide variety of federal and state laws, as well as payor program requirements, may not have the time to acquire that understanding. He or she will rely on technology specialists, perhaps the organization's IT staff or outside experts. The section that follows is an overview of the individual security measures mandated by HIPAA.

ADMINISTRATIVE SAFEGUARDS

The administrative safeguards are concerned with the institutional structures that ensure the security and integrity of E-PHI.

Security Management Process Standard. A covered entity must identify and analyze potential risks to E-PHI, and implement security measures that reduce risks and vulnerabilities to a reasonable and appropriate level. It accomplishes this through these four specifications.

The required *Risk Analysis* and *Risk Management* specifications were described earlier in the chapter. Risk management is the program that a covered entity follows to minimize the risks identified by the risk analysis. The entity must institute a *Sanction Policy* that applies appropriate sanctions against workforce members who fail to comply with its security policies and procedures. Under the *Information System Activity Review* specification, a covered entity is required to implement procedures to regularly review records of information system activity, such as audit logs, access reports, and security incident tracking reports.

Assigned Security Responsibility Standard. A covered entity must designate a security official who is responsible for developing and implementing its security policies and procedures. Beyond this statement, there is no implementation specification.

Workforce Security Standard. Covered entities must ensure that all their employees have appropriate access to E-PHI and that employees who lack access authorization are not able to gain access to E-PHI. They can do this by implementing three specifications.

The entities must implement *Authorization and Supervision* of employees who work with E-PHI. They also must institute a *Workforce Clearance Procedure* that ensures that employees working with E-PHI have appropriate access. Finally, there must be a *Termination Procedure* that cuts off E-PHI access when an employee leaves the organization.

Information Access Management Standard. Consistent with the Privacy Rule limit on uses and disclosures of PHI to the "minimum necessary," the Security Rule requires a covered entity to implement policies and procedures for authorizing access to E-PHI only when it is appropriate to the user's job duties. This is accomplished through three specifications.

If the covered entity is a healthcare clearinghouse that is part of a larger organization, it must install policies and procedures to *Isolate the E-PHI of the Clearinghouse* from the rest of the organization. The entity should implement policies and procedures for *Authorizing Access* to E-PHI. This should be complemented by *Access Establishment and Modification* policies and procedures that establish, document, review, and modify a user's right of access.

Security Awareness and Training Standard. This standard requires that covered entities implement a security and awareness training program for all its employees, including management. There are four implementation specifications.

A covered entity should regularly issue *Security Reminders* of its security policies and procedures. It should implement measures that provide *Protection from Malicious Software*. There should be procedures in effect for *Monitoring Log-In Attempts* and reporting discrepancies. The entity also should maintain procedures for *Password Management*, creating, changing, and safeguarding them.

Security Incident Procedures Standard. This crucial standard asks covered entities to implement policies and procedures to address "security incidents," which are defined as "the attempted or successful unauthorized access, use, disclosure, modification, or destruction of information or interference with system operations in an information system." The single implementation specification under this standard requires that the entities *Identify and Respond* to the incidents, take action to mitigate their harmful effects, and document the final outcomes.

Contingency Plan Standard. Here, covered entities must establish policies and procedures for dealing with an emergency or other occurrence (fire, vandalism, system failure, or natural disaster) that could damage systems that contain E-PHI. There are five implementation specifications that contribute to this goal.

A covered entity must implement procedures to:

1. Create and maintain retrievable exact copies of E-PHI (*Data Backup Plan*).
2. Restore any loss of data (*Disaster Recovery Plan*).
3. Enable continuation of critical business processes for protecting E-PHI security during an emergency (*Emergency Mode Operation Plan*).

4. Periodically test and revise contingency plans (*Testing and Revision Procedure*).
5. Assess the relative criticality of specific applications and data in support of the other contingency plan elements (*Applications and Data Criticality Analysis*).

Evaluation Standard. This standard calls upon covered entities to perform a periodic assessment of how well their security policies and procedures meet the requirements of the Security Rule.

PHYSICAL SAFEGUARDS

Facility Access Controls Standard. A covered entity must limit physical access to its electronic information systems and the facilities where they are located, while also ensuring that authorized access is allowed. It will accomplish this by means of four specifications.

In conjunction with the *Contingency Plan Standard* (administrative safeguards), covered entities must develop a procedure to allow *Facility Access* in support of restoration of lost data under the disaster recovery plan and emergency mode operations plan in the event of an emergency. They also must create a *Facility Security Plan* that safeguards the facility and the equipment inside from unauthorized physical access, tampering, or theft. The law requires that covered entities implement *Access Control and Validation Procedures* that manage employee access to facilities based on their work responsibilities. This includes access to software programs and control of visitors to the premises. The entities have an obligation to document repairs and modifications to the security-related components of their facilities (*Maintenance Records*).

Workstation Use Standard. This standard deals with the functions to be performed at E-PHI accessible workstations, the manner in which the functions will be performed, and the physical surroundings of each type of workstation. There is no implementation specification for this standard.

Workstation Security Standard. Under this standard, covered entities must implement physical safeguards for all E-PHI accessible workstations to restrict access to authorized users. There is no further specification for this standard.

Device and Media Controls Standard. Each covered entity must put into place policies and procedures that govern the movement of hardware and electronic media containing E-PHI into and out of a facility, and within the facility. There are four implementation specifications to guide this effort.

The entity must create policies and procedures that address:

1. The final disposition of E-PHI and the media on which it is stored (*Disposal*).
2. The removal of E-PHI from electronic media before they are reused (*Media Reuse*).
3. The maintenance of a record of the movements of hardware and electronic media (*Accountability*).
4. The creation of a retrievable, exact copy of E-PHI before equipment is moved (*Data Backup and Storage*).

TECHNICAL SAFEGUARDS

Access Control Standard. The purpose of this standard is to allow access to E-PHI systems only to those persons or computer applications that have been granted access rights under the *Information Access Management Standard*. Four specifications have been defined for accomplishing this.

First, the covered entity must assign a unique name or number for identifying and tracking user identity. Second, it must establish procedures for obtaining needed E-PHI during an emergency. Third, it must set up procedures that terminate a computer session after a specified period of inactivity. Fourth, the entity must implement a mechanism to encrypt and decrypt E-PHI.

Audit Controls Standard. This standard requires that covered entities implement hardware, software, or procedural mechanisms that record and examine activity in computer systems that contain E-PHI. No implementation specification is provided.

Integrity Controls Standard. The goal of this standard is to protect E-PHI from improper alteration or destruction. Each covered entity is asked to implement *Electronic Mechanisms to Confirm* that no E-PHI has been altered or destroyed in an unauthorized manner.

Person or Entity Authentication Standard. Covered entities must institute measures to verify that a person or entity seeking access to their E-PHI are who they claim to be. There is no implementation specification here.

Transmission Security Standard. The function of this standard is to guard against unauthorized access to E-PHI that is being transmitted over an electronic network. There are two specifications.

One requires *Integrity Controls* to ensure that the E-PHI is not improperly modified without detection before it is discarded. The other calls for *Encryption* of E-PHI whenever it is appropriate.

ENFORCEMENT OF THE PRIVACY RULE

The HIPAA states that the DHHS will seek the cooperation of covered entities in complying voluntarily with the Privacy Rule. Failing that, the OCR within DHHS will enforce the Rule through civil monetary and criminal penalties. All these penalties can also be imposed on business associates.

Civil monetary penalties. The DHHS may impose civil monetary penalties (CMP) on a covered entity of at least $100 per failure to comply with a HIPAA requirement. There are four tiers of penalties reflecting increasing levels of culpability. They work like this.
1. Violations that the covered entity did not know about and could not have known about with "reasonable diligence." Each violation: $100–$50,000
2. Violations for which there was "reasonable cause" but no "willful neglect." Each violation: $1,000–$50,000
3. Violations caused by willful neglect that are corrected within 30 days. Each violation: $10,000–$50,000
4. Violations caused by willful neglect that are not corrected within 30 days. Each violation: $50,000–$50,000

At all four levels, the maximum total penalties imposed for identical violations during a single calendar year is $1,500,000.

Reasonable diligence is defined as "the business care and prudence expected from a person seeking to satisfy a legal requirement under similar circumstances." *Reasonable cause* is defined as "circumstances that make it unreasonable for the covered entity, despite the exercise of ordinary business care and prudence, to comply with the administrative simplification provision violated." *Willful neglect* is defined as the "conscious, intentional failure or reckless indifference to the obligation to comply with the administrative simplification provision violated."

The new CMPs are in addition to and not in lieu of any fines and penalties that a state might impose. State Attorneys General are also empowered to bring civil actions under HIPAA.

Criminal penalties. A person who knowingly obtains or discloses individually identifiable health information in violation of HIPAA faces a fine of $50,000 and up to 1 year of imprisonment. The criminal penalties increase to $100,000 and up to 5 years imprisonment if the wrongful conduct involves false pretenses, and to $250,000 and up to 10 years imprisonment if the wrongful conduct involves the intent to sell, transfer, or use individually identifiable health information for commercial advantage, personal gain, or malicious harm.

The HITECH Act requires DHHS to carry out periodic audits to ensure covered entities and business associates are complying with the HIPAA Privacy and Security Rules and Breach Notification standards. Beginning in November 2011 and concluding in December 2012, the OCR conducted a pilot program that performed 115 audits of covered entities to assess their privacy and security compliance.

CASE EXAMPLES OF HIPAA ENFORCEMENT

In September 2012, the *Massachusetts Eye and Ear Infirmary* agreed to pay the DHHS $1.5 million to settle potential violations of the HIPAA Privacy and Security Rules. The Infirmary has also agreed to take corrective action to improve policies and procedures to safeguard the privacy and security of their patients' PHI and retain an independent monitor to report on its compliance efforts. The OCR conducted an investigation following a breach report submitted by the Infirmary, as required by the HIPAA Breach Notification Rule, reporting the theft of an unencrypted personal laptop containing the E-PHI of patients and research subjects. The information included patient prescriptions and clinical information. The investigation showed that while management was aware of the Security Rule, the Infirmary failed to take necessary steps to comply with the Rule's requirements, such as conducting a thorough analysis of the risk to the confidentiality of E-PHI maintained on portable devices; implementing security measures sufficient to ensure the confidentiality of E-PHI that was created, maintained, and transmitted using portable devices; adopting and implementing policies and procedures to restrict access to E-PHI to authorized users of portable devices; and adopting and implementing policies and procedures to address security incident identification, reporting, and response.

In April 2012, *Phoenix Cardiac Surgery* agreed to pay DHHS a $100,000 settlement amount and implement a corrective action plan that includes a review of recently developed policies and other actions taken to come into full compliance with the Privacy and Security Rules. OCR's investigation found that the physician practice was posting clinical and surgical appointments for their patients on an Internet-based calendar that was publicly accessible. In addition, Phoenix Cardiac Surgery had implemented few policies and procedures to comply with the HIPAA Privacy and Security Rules, and had limited safeguards in place to protect patients' E-PHI.

INCORPORATING HIPAA/HITECH COMPLIANCE INTO THE OVERALL ORGANIZATIONAL COMPLIANCE PROGRAM

Compliance with HIPAA and HITECH requirements is a different matter than complying with laws like the False Claims Act and the Anti-Kickback Statute. HIPAA violations rarely are intentional or lead to overpayments and distortions in the healthcare system. Computer systems and electronic data transmission are pervasive features throughout healthcare delivery and financing. Their role will only grow in the future. Nonetheless, there are serious legal implications for ignoring HIPAA.

There are two general ways to approach HIPAA compliance. Because of its technological complexity, some organizations, usually larger entities with more resources, may prefer to create HIPAA compliance programs separate from the traditional fraud and abuse compliance activities they already conduct. On the other hand, it may make more sense for smaller, less well-endowed organizations, like physician practices or billing companies, to combine the two. In that second case, it will be necessary to hire or contract with someone with the necessary computer expertise.

The HIPAA and HITECH laws and regulations provide far more detail about how covered entities must manage their electronic data systems and the PHI that they use and transmit. Some of the standards and specifications overlap each other. The DHHS has shown flexibility in what it will accept as satisfactory compliance by healthcare organizations. In one form or another, every covered entity must carry out these steps.

- Designate a HIPAA compliance or patient privacy official.
- Write and put into practice the numerous policies and procedures called for in the standards and specifications.
- Train all members of the workforce on the HIPAA privacy requirements.
- Develop and apply sanctions to employees for violations of the privacy policies and procedures.
- Communicate with patients about their privacy rights and how to complain about privacy violations.
- Maintain a record of all actions, activities, and assessments that are required to be documented by the Security Rule.

There is a multipage explanation of an excellent HIPAA compliance program at the website of the University of Texas at San Antonio: http://www.uthscsa.edu/hipaa/.

STUDY QUESTIONS

1. What is the difference between the Privacy Rule and the Security Rule? How does each support and interact with the other?
2. Why is the HIPAA Security Rule needed and what is the purpose of the security standards?
3. Why is the HIPAA Privacy Rule needed?
4. When can a healthcare organization use or disclose a patient's PHI without the patient's permission?
5. Explain the "minimum necessary" rule of PHI use and disclosure.
6. When you are a patient in a hospital, what are your rights regarding the information that the hospital collects about you?
7. Explain in detail the "breach" to which the Breach Notification Rule applies.
8. After you have read through the Security Rule standards in all three safeguard categories, which of them do you understand well enough to implement (through policies and procedures) on your own? For which of them would you need some expert assistance?
9. List 10 types of organizations that are considered to be "covered entities" by HIPAA. What is a "healthcare clearinghouse"?

Learning Exercises

1. Choose one of these three standards (Security Incident Procedures, Workforce Security, Facility Access Controls) and prepare a 1-page written procedure that implements it.

2. Watch news reports closely and notice the next time that a breach of PHI is announced. They happen with surprising frequency. Read all you can about the incident and the organization where it happened. Get an idea of what led to the breach. What appears to have gone wrong? How could the incident have been prevented?

3. Describe five steps that a physician practice should take after it discovers that one of its staff has accessed the PHI of a local celebrity being treated by the practice and shared it with some of his or her friends.

4. Draw up a form that patients would be required to sign authorizing a covered entity to share their PHI with a research project being conducted within the entity.

5. In the course of enforcing HIPAA, the OCR has answered many questions raised by covered entities, business associates, patients, and others affected by the law. You can go to this webpage and, by entering a few keywords, gain access to the answers provided to questions about most aspects of the HIPAA law and regulations: http://www.hhs.gov/ocr/privacy/hipaa/faq/index.html.

REFERENCES

1. Summary of the HIPAA Security Rule, DHHS, http://www.hhs.gov/ocr/privacy/hipaa/understanding/srsummary.html
2. Summary of the HIPAA Privacy Rule, DHHS, http://www.hhs.gov/ocr/privacy/hipaa/understanding/summary/index.html
3. Summary of the HIPAA Privacy Rule, OCR Privacy Brief, Department of Health and Human Services, Office for Civil Rights, May 2003.
4. HIPAA Administrative Simplification Statute and Rules, OCR, http://www.hhs.gov/ocr/privacy/hipaa/administrative/index.html
5. HIPAA Administrative Simplification: Enforcement, Federal Register, Vol. 74, No. 209, October 30, 2009.
6. Covered Entity, Business Associate, and Organizational Options, OCR PowerPoint presentation, Feb/Mar 2003, http://www.hhs.gov/ocr/privacy/hipaa/understanding/training/coveredentities.pdf
7. Protected Health Information, Uses and Disclosures, and Minimum Necessary, OCR PowerPoint presentation, Feb/Mar 2003, http://www.hhs.gov/ocr/privacy/hipaa/understanding/training/udmn.pdf
8. Administrative Requirements, OCR PowerPoint presentation, Feb/Mar 2003, http://www.hhs.gov/ocr/privacy/hipaa/understanding/training/adminreq.pdf
9. Compliance and Enforcement, OCR PowerPoint presentation, Feb/Mar 2003, http://www.hhs.gov/ocr/privacy/hipaa/understanding/training/compli.pdf

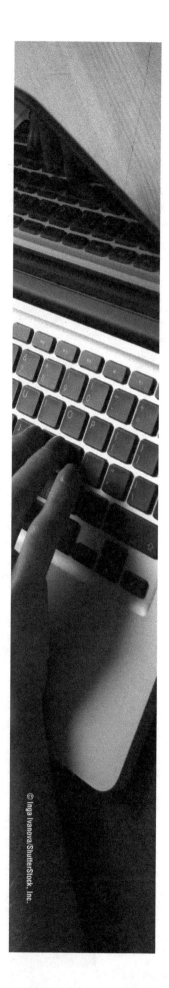

Privacy, Confidentiality, Security, and Integrity of Electronic Data

Objectives

Discuss the concepts of privacy, confidentiality, security, and integrity as they apply to the management of electronic data.

Recognize common threats to the privacy, confidentiality, security, and integrity of data that electronic systems encompass and store.

Apply effective procedures for protecting data, software, and hardware.

Follow Health Insurance Portability and Accountability Act (HIPAA) principles for protecting healthcare information.

Discuss healthcare security issues as they relate to the Internet and the role of healthcare providers in protecting patient data.

Introduction

This chapter identifies threats to privacy and confidentiality as well as threats to integrity and security of information. Privacy refers to a person's desire to limit the disclosure of personal information. Confidentiality deals with the healthcare provider's responsibility to limit access to information so that it is shared in a controlled manner for the benefit of the patient. Security refers to the measures that organizations implement to protect information and systems. Integrity refers to the accuracy and comprehensiveness of data.

The code of ethics for healthcare professionals consistently demonstrates that ensuring the confidentiality and privacy of patient, client, and consumer information is a major responsibility of healthcare providers. Meeting that responsibility is impossible if the healthcare provider does not understand how to follow current regulations and apply effective procedures for protecting electronic data. These issues are even more of a concern with the advent of social media sites used by healthcare professionals. This chapter clarifies the regulations for protecting healthcare information. In addition, healthcare providers are responsible for ensuring the security and integrity of patient data; this chapter describes procedures for protecting data, software, and hardware.

Using Computer Systems for Storing Data

With rare exceptions, all healthcare institutions manage and store data in automated systems. These data, which relate to clients, employees, and the institution, are interrelated and interdependent. A threat to any data element in these automated systems can be a threat to the clients, the employees, and the institution. The legal and ethical implications related to storing personal health-related data are of primary concern.

Concerns with confidentiality and security are not limited to healthcare information systems. Many personal computers and mobile devices now store or access significant confidential data. Stolen data from these personal systems can be a major source of problems. Identity theft occurs when a person takes someone's identifying information and uses it for fraudulent purposes. There are several different types of identity theft. These are the most common:

- Medical identity theft occurs when someone uses another person's personal information with or without that individual's knowledge or consent to obtain healthcare and/or receive payment for such care. Victims of medical identity theft may discover that their medical records are inaccurate. This inaccuracy is not only medically dangerous for the victim, but can also affect his or her ability to obtain insurance coverage or benefits (Federal Trade Commission, 2012a).
- Child identity theft occurs when identity thieves use a child's Social Security number. For example, the child's identity may be used to apply for government benefits, open bank and credit card accounts, or rent a place to live (Federal Trade Commission, 2012b).
- Tax-related identity theft occurs when someone uses a person's Social Security number to obtain a job or to steal a tax refund.

The different types of identity theft often overlap. For example, someone may use a child's Social Security number to obtain a job, medical care, or Social Security payments. An intake history or nursing assessment may pick up warning signs of identity theft. If a patient provides a health history that includes information that is not congruent with previous medical records or comments on medical bills for services never received, the provider should investigate these types of incongruences.

Concerns with data integrity and security are not limited to healthcare or personal data. Most files on a computer represent hours of work that can be very difficult to replicate. For example, if a student spent several hours completing a term paper that a computer virus destroys, it may be difficult to convince the instructor that a virus "ate the paper."

Five major concerns arise in conjunction with electronically stored data, whether it is stored on a healthcare information system, on an Internet server, or on a personal computer:

- Providing for privacy and confidentiality of data.
- Ensuring the integrity of the data.
- Protecting hardware and devices as well as the software and apps that are used to manage and store these data.
- To the extent possible, minimizing the impact of the lost or destroyed data.
- Recognizing and prosecuting criminal abuse of computer data and equipment.

Privacy and Confidentiality

To protect privacy and confidentiality, you must address issues relevant to data storage and use. Problems of ensuring privacy and confidentiality of data include data protection issues and data integrity issues. Data protection issues include accessing data for unauthorized use and unnecessary storage of data. Data integrity issues include incomplete or inaccurate data and intentional or accidental manipulation of data.

Personal Privacy and Confidentiality

With the advent of computers, numerous companies, institutions, and government agencies maintain databases containing personal data. For example, personal information related to education, including learning disabilities and financial need data, is stored on university computers. The Department of Motor Vehicles stores personal driving record information; the Social Security Administration stores Social Security benefits information; and retail companies store personal information such as phone numbers, addresses, and items that customers have ordered as well as credit card numbers. Insurance companies maintain extensive information on their customers' personal health care. Knowing what data others are storing is an important first step in protecting individual privacy.

When individuals complete warranty or registration forms that ask for their names, addresses, and other information, companies can collect and sell these data to other companies. Simply using the Internet generates information about individuals—where they go on the Internet, who they interact with via social media sites, and which products they buy. Several organizations have evolved to respond to online privacy issues; **Table** 1 lists several of these

TABLE 1	ORGANIZATIONS PROTECTING ONLINE PRIVACY	
Name	URL	Description
Center for Democracy and Technology (CDT)	http://www.cdt.org/	CDT is a 501(c)(3) nonprofit public policy organization founded in 1994 to promote democratic values and constitutional liberties. Areas of focus include: preserving the open, decentralized, and user-controlled nature of the Internet; enhancing freedom of expression; protecting privacy; and limiting government surveillance.
Center for Democracy and Technology (CDT)—Health Privacy	https://www.cdt.org /issue/health-privacy	In March 2008, CDT launched an initiative to address the complex privacy issues associated with the use of health information technology.
Electronic Privacy Information Center (EPIC)	http://epic.org/	EPIC is a 501(c)(3) nonprofit public interest research center established in 1994 to focus public attention on emerging civil liberties issues and to protect privacy, the First Amendment, and constitutional values.
Privacy International (PI)	http://www .privacyinternational .org/	PI, formed in 1990, is registered in the UK as a charity focused on defending the right to privacy across the world by fighting unlawful surveillance and intrusions into private life by governments and corporations.
Electronic Frontier Foundation (EFF)	http://www.eff.org/	EFF, founded in 1990, focuses on defending free speech, privacy, innovation, and consumer digital rights. EFF's primary approach is in the courts—bringing and defending lawsuits.
Privacy Rights Clearinghouse (PRC)	http://www .privacyrights.org/	PRC is a California 501(c)(3) nonprofit established in 1992 focused on consumer information and consumer advocacy. For example, it works to raise consumers' awareness of how technology affects privacy and empowers consumers to control access to their personal information.

organizations. Notice that each of these organizations was established in the early 1990s, just as the Internet was becoming available to the general public. While each of these groups takes a different approach to protecting online privacy, all include education of the public as one of their approaches. For example, The Privacy Rights Clearinghouse (https://www.privacyrights.org/privacy-rights-fact-sheets) has more than 50 fact sheets, including a group specific to the privacy of personal health data. Each fact sheet deals with a different online privacy topic. For example, Fact Sheet 21 is a resource guide for dealing with children's online privacy (Privacy Rights Clearinghouse, 2012a).

Currently, many organizations share personal data from their databases. By sharing information across these databases, it becomes possible to create a personal profile of an individual that is more extensive than you might imagine. For example, you should read the small print privacy statements on leaflets that are mailed with credit bills or bank statements. The Medical Information Board/ MIB Group, Inc. (MIB) provides another excellent example within health care. MIB is an association of approximately 475 U.S. and Canadian life and health insurance companies. By sharing information, these companies work together to ensure the consistency of health information that they collect during the insurance application process (MIB, n.d.). MIB provides free access to individuals requesting a copy of their files. Since many people do not know they have a record with MIB, few checks and balances exist to ensure the accuracy of this information. For example, a company may refuse to offer an individual life insurance and the individual may never know that the reason for the refusal was the presence of inaccurate information in the MIB file.

Patient Privacy and Confidentiality

Because many people believe that the information they share with their healthcare providers is held in confidence, they may assume a level of protection that does not exist. Once the related medical record includes that information, however, the actual confidentiality of that information is determined by who has access to those data. Healthcare information is shared not only with physicians, nurses, and other healthcare providers, but also with insurance companies and government agencies such as Medicare or Medicaid. Others obtain legal access to these records when individuals agree to let others see them, usually by signing consent forms when receiving health care.

HIPAA, which is discussed in more detail later in this chapter, establishes federal privacy standards for medical records that healthcare providers, health plans, and health clearinghouses maintain. However, a great deal of health-related information exists *outside* of healthcare facilities and their business partners and, therefore, is beyond the reach of HIPAA. This includes employee files, school records, and organizations such as MIB. Under both the HIPAA and the Patriot Act, there are certain circumstances when police may access medical records without a warrant (Burke & Weill, 2005). Although HIPAA requires that others inform you about how they may use your records without your consent, it does not require that others inform you when your records are actually shared. In addition, the Patriot Act includes provisions that prohibit notifying you if others share your medical records under the provisions of this act.

> *Under Section 215 of the Patriot Act, the Federal Government has the authority to request (i) a court order requiring a physician to produce medical records ("production order"), as well as (ii) a concurrently issued non-disclosure order ("gag order") that prohibits a physician from disclosing to any other person (except for an attorney or persons necessary for compliance with the production order) the existence of the production order* (American Medical Association, 2007).

Data Integrity Concepts

Ensuring patient privacy is necessary but not sufficient for ensuring patient safety. If the collected and processed data for providing patient care lacks integrity, the resulting care will be dangerously inadequate. Data are uninterpreted facts or observations that describe an event or phenomenon. Data integrity refers to the truthfulness and accuracy of the data. For example, one might describe a patient's weight as 130 lbs. If the patient's weight is actually 150 lbs., the data is of poor quality or inaccurate. Providers and information systems process data to produce information and are therefore the foundation for effective healthcare decisions and critical thinking. The following list of principles is the result of work by American Health Information Management Association (2007) and provides examples of appropriate data integrity maintenance in healthcare records:

- Access permissions are in accordance with clear written policies that enforce and that ensure only the appropriately educated healthcare personal can create, read, update, and delete data from any healthcare-related records.
- A data dictionary is created, maintained, and used. The data dictionary includes standardized data field definitions for each data element. For example, nursing diagnoses used in the patients' health records follow a clearly defined standardized language.
- A standardized data entry and processing format is used to ensure consistency. This includes standardized data entry screens as well as the process for entering data.
- Laws, regulations, accreditation standards, and standards of practice are reinforced and incorporated into all aspects of the data entry process.
- Data integrity policies and procedures are developed and followed. For example, different departments should not maintain a separate list of patient allergies. Rather, the patient's record should include one comprehensive list that is used by all departments.

Safety and Security

Protecting the safety and security of patient data involves identifying threats to computer systems and initiating procedures to protect the integrity of the data and system. The two main types of threats are related to the integrity of data and to the confidentiality of the data. These threats can result from accidental or intentional human actions or natural disasters. Destruction of data, hardware, and software by natural disasters include damage by water, fire, earthquakes, or chemicals; electrical power outages; disk failures; and exposure to magnetic fields. The types of human actions that result in these threats fall into five areas: innocent mistakes, inappropriate access by insiders for curiosity reasons, inappropriate access by insiders for spite or for profit, unauthorized intruders who gain access to patient data, and vengeful employees and outsiders (National Academy of Sciences, 1997).

Innocent Mistakes

Innocent mistakes are errors made by people who have legal access to the system and who, in the process of using the system, accidentally disclose data or damage the integrity of data. Examples can be as simple as a healthcare provider recording data in the wrong medical record or a lab sending a fax to the wrong fax number. In school, it may take the form of a teacher entering the wrong grade on the student's academic record. M. Eric Johnson documented several incidences of accidental disclosure of medical data in a paper titled "Data Hemorrhages in a Health Care Sector." Examples given in this paper include: accidentally posting medical data to the Internet such as occurred when the Wuesthoff Medical Center in Florida posted information on more than 500 patients; the Tampa-based WellCare Health Plans posted information on 71,000 Georgia residents; and the University of Pittsburgh Medical Center posted names and medical images of nearly 80 individuals (Johnson, 2009). Additional case examples of HIPAA Resolution Agreements can be viewed at http://www.hhs.gov/ocr/privacy/hipaa/enforcement/examples/index.html.

Inappropriate Access by Insiders for Curiosity Reasons

Sometimes people with legal access to the system make an intentional decision to abuse their access privileges. Browsing is a problem with many electronic record systems—and health records are not immune to this problem. In this type of access, the person looks at medical records for the express purpose of satisfying his or her own curiosity or goals; the access to the medical record provides no benefit to the patient. The auditing functions in many healthcare information systems, however, make it easy to identify these browsers and discipline those individuals. **Table** 2 includes several current examples of employees who

TABLE 2 EXAMPLES OF EMPLOYEES FIRED FOR INAPPROPRIATE ACCESS OF MEDICAL RECORDS

News Source and Date of Publication	Headline	URL
PHIprivacy.net December 21, 2012 2:30 P.M.	CCS Medical employee may have accessed and disclosed Social Security numbers for a tax refund fraud scheme	http://www.phiprivacy.net/?p=11056
MSN News Canada July 25, 2012 16:58:18	5 employees fired after Eastern Health privacy breaches	http://news.ca.msn.com/canada /5-employees-fired-after-eastern-health -privacy-breaches
HeraldNet March 14, 2012, 12:01 A.M.	Everett Clinic fires 13 for snooping	http://heraldnet.com/article/20120314 /NEWS01/703149862
New4Jax October 14, 2011 11:59:07 A.M.	20 Hospital Workers Fired for Viewing Collier's Medical Records	http://www.news4jax.com /news/20-Hospital-Workers-Fired -for-Viewing-Collier-s-Medical -Records/-/475880/2062868/-/r6ctbjz /-/index.html
Huffington Post Media Group: NCAAF Sporting News February 3, 2011 at 2:30 P.M.	Iowa hospital employees fired over Hawkeyes' medical records breaches	http://aol.sportingnews.com/ncaa -football/story/2011-02-03/iowa-hospital -employees-fired-over-hawkeyes-medical -records-breaches
Arizona Daily Star January 12, 2011	3 UMC workers fired for records access	http://azstarnet.com/news/local/crime /umc-workers-fired-for-records-access /article_4f789a48-1e8c-11e0-929a -001cc4c002e0.html

were fired for this very reason. In educational institutions, browsing an academic record without an academic purpose is a clear violation of Family Educational Rights and Privacy Act (FERPA) regulations.

Inappropriate Access by Insiders for Spite or for Profit

Healthcare professionals play an important role in protecting patients from exploitation for personal or financial gain. Such violations damage the reputation of an institution and can be expensive. Recently, UCLA paid a fine of $865,500 in a settlement reached between the U.S. Department of Health and Human

Services (HHS) and the University of California at Los Angeles Health System (UCLA Health Center) over a breach of patient records (HHS, 2011). News stories reported that multiple internal employees over many years had improperly accessed the medical records of several high-profile/celebrity patients. Neither HHS nor UCLA confirmed the names of the celebrities but media reports have mentioned many of these celebrities (Jenkins, 2011).

Farrah Fawcett, who was a patient under treatment for cancer at UCLA during this period, set up her own sting to prove to UCLA that someone at their health center was leaking her medical information. After information known only to Fawcett and her doctor was quickly leaked to the *National Enquirer*, UCLA investigated. The Institution found that one employee had accessed her records more often than her own doctors. This woman pleaded guilty to a single count of violating federal medical privacy law for commercial purposes, but died of cancer before she could be sentenced (Ornstein, 2009).

Unauthorized Intruders Who Gain Access to Patient Data

Many hospitals rely on physical security, software, and user education to protect the information stored inside a computer from unauthorized intruders. For example, hospitals may locate the computers where it is difficult for others to access or use them. Hospitals may also use passwords and firewalls to control access. In addition, hospitals may set computers to automatically log off users after a few minutes of inactivity.

Vengeful Employees and Outsiders

Examples of data incursions by vengeful individuals include vindictive patients or intruders who mount attacks to access unauthorized information or damage systems and disrupt operations. For this reason, most hospitals terminate an employee's computer access before informing the employee of the termination and physically escort the terminated employee off the premises.

Examples of additional reported HIPAA violations can be located at:

- https://www.privacyrights.org/data-breach/new
- http://www.phiprivacy.net/
- http://www.hhs.gov/ocr/privacy/hipaa/administrative/breachnotificationrule/breachtool.html

Computer Crime

Computer crimes include a wide range of illegal activities, from computer intrusion into a computer system (i.e., hacking) to child pornography or exploitation. Some of these crimes require a certain level of technical skill, but many are as simple as sending an email with false or misleading information. An individual may perpetrate such crimes; large organized crime groups and even governments may carry out other such crimes. Victims range from vulnerable individuals or organizations to corporations and government institutions that are vital to the infrastructure of the country.

Like many tough issues, cybersecurity is a cross-cutting problem, affecting not only all Federal agencies, but also state and local governments, the private sector, non-governmental organizations, academia, and other countries. It is a national security, homeland security, economic security, network defense, and law enforcement issue all rolled into one (Daniel, 2012).

As a result, several government agencies are involved in investigating these types of crimes. **Table** 3 lists several of these agencies, their URLs, and their missions.

TABLE 3 GOVERNMENT AND GOVERNMENT-RELATED AGENCIES PREVENTING AND PROSECUTING COMPUTER CRIMES		
Agency	URL	Mission
Computer Crime & Intellectual Property Section United States Department of Justice (CCIPS)	http://www.justice.gov /criminal/cybercrime/	Responsible for implementing the Department's national strategies in combating computer and intellectual property crimes worldwide including electronic penetrations, data thefts, and cyber-attacks on critical information systems.
FBI: Cyber Crime Division	http://www.fbi.gov /about-us/investigate /cyber/cyber	Investigates high-tech crimes, including cyber-based terrorism, espionage, computer intrusions, and major cyberfraud.
Federal Trade Commission (FTC) Bureau of Consumer Protection	http://www.ftc.gov/bcp /index.shtml	Prevents and investigates business practices that are anticompetitive, deceptive, or unfair to consumers including computer and Internet-related practices.
National Security Council: Cybersecurity	http://www.whitehouse .gov/administration/eop /nsc/cybersecurity	Leads the interagency development of national cybersecurity strategy and policy and oversees the agencies' implementation of those policies.
Internet Crime Complaint Center (IC3)	http://www.ic3.gov /default.aspx	Partnership between the Federal Bureau of Investigation (FBI), the National White Collar Crime Center (NW3C), and the Bureau of Justice Assistance (BJA). IC3's mission is to serve as a vehicle to receive, develop, and refer criminal complaints regarding the rapidly expanding arena of cybercrime.

TABLE	3	(CONTINUED)	
National White Collar Crime Center (NW3C)	http://www.nw3c.org/	A congressionally funded, nonprofit corporation whose mission is to provide training, investigative support, and research to agencies and entities involved in the prevention, investigation, and prosecution of economic and high-tech crime.	
United States Postal Inspection Service (USPIS)	http://postalinspectors .uspis.gov/	Investigates crimes dealing with mail fraud involving both postal mail services and the Internet.	
United States Secret Service: Electronic Crimes Task Forces and Working Groups	http://www .secretservice .gov/ectf.shtml	Provides the necessary support and resources to investigate economic crimes that meet one of the following criteria: • Significant economic or community impact • Participation of organized criminal groups involving multiple districts or transnational organizations • Use of schemes involving new technology.	

As computer crime has evolved, so have the language and terms used to discuss these crimes. **Table** 4 defines a number of these terms as well as a few data protection terms.

TABLE	4	TERMS RELATED TO COMPUTER CRIME
Term		Definition
Adware		A type of software that downloads or displays unwanted advertisements on a computer.
Cracker		A hacker that illegally breaks into computer systems and creates mischief.
Cybercrime		The use of the Internet or other communication technology to commit a crime of any type.
Data Diddling		Modifying valid data in a computer file.
Denial of Service		Any action or series of actions that prevents any part of an information system from functioning. For example, using several computers attached to the Internet to access a Web site so that the site is overwhelmed and not available.
Encryption		Method of coding sensitive data to protect it when sent over the Internet.
Firewall		A software program used to protect computers from unauthorized access via the Iinternet.

(continues)

TABLE 4	TERMS RELATED TO COMPUTER CRIME (continued)
Hacker	Originally a compulsive computer programmer, it now has a more negative meaning and is often confused with "cracker."
Identity Theft	When someone uses another person's private information to assume their identity.
Keyboard Loggers	Hardware or software installed on a computer to log the keystrokes of an individual. A keyboard logger can be used to monitor computer activities such as time spent on the linternet or collect personal information such as passwords.
Logic Bomb	Piece of program code buried within another program, designed to perform some malicious act in response to a trigger. The trigger can involve entering data or a name, for example.
Malware	General term used to refer to viruses, worms, spyware, Trojan Horses, and adware.
Opt-out	A number of measures to prevent receiving unwanted products or services. For example, if you sign up for a free journal on the Internet you may want to opt-out of receiving emails and product announcements from companies that advertise in this journal. In many cases the default is that you opt-in.
Phishing	(Pronounced *fishing*.) Creating a replica of a legitimate Web page to hook users and trick them into submitting personal or financial information or passwords.
Sabotage	The purposeful destruction of hardware, software, or data.
Salami Method	A method of data stealing that involves taking little bits at a time.
Software Piracy	Unauthorized copying of copyrighted software.
Spamming	The act of sending unsolicited electronic messages in bulk.
Theft of Services	The unauthorized use of services such as a computer system.
Time Bomb	Instructions in a program that perform certain functions on a specific date or time such as printing a message or destroying data.
Trapdoors	Methods installed by programmers that allow unauthorized access to programs.
Trojan Horse	Placing instructions in a program that add additional, illegitimate functions; for example, the program prints out information every time information on a certain patient is entered.
Virus	A program that, once introduced into a system, replicates itself and causes a variety of mischievous outcomes. Viruses are usually introduced from infected USB storage devices, email attachments, and downloaded files.
Worm	A destructive program that can fill various memory locations of a computer system with information, clogging the system so that other operations are compromised.

Prosecution of Computer Crime

It is difficult to detect and persecute many computer crimes. Many times, the person initiating the criminal act does not live in this country and may not be subject to U.S. laws. The U.S. Department of Justice maintains a key resource for understanding computer crime and related issues; this website can be found at http://www.justice .gov/usao/briefing_room/cc/index.html. Although the terms in Table   4 are more readily identified with computer crime in areas other than health care, all types of crimes can and do occur within healthcare computer systems.

Some computer crimes are detected but not reported. When data are stolen, the information is not always seen as valuable; thus those responsible for its theft may not be prosecuted. Many times, an institution will be more concerned with the poor publicity that can result from disclosure of this event. However, the breach notification provision of HIPAA required notification of patients using criteria outlined in HIPAA. These criteria were strengthened in January 2013 with the implementation of the Health Information Technology for Economic and Clinical Health (HITECH) breach notification requirements, which clarifies when breaches of unsecured health information must be reported to HHS and to patients. Additional information concerning these requirements can be seen at http://www.hhs.gov/ocr/privacy/hipaa/administrative/omnibus/index.html.

Although methods for tracking entry into computer systems are becoming increasingly sophisticated, discovery of computer crime may be difficult. Laws are catching up, but still lag behind computer technology. In some situations, there are questions about who "owns" data. Therefore, early laws in this area protected individuals from having data about them stored in a computer without their knowledge.

Selected Laws Related to Computing

Freedom of Information Act of 1970: This law allows citizens to have access to data gathered by federal agencies.

Federal Privacy Act of 1974: This law stipulates that there can be no secret personal files; individuals must be allowed to know what is stored in files about them and how it is used. This act applies to government agencies and contractors dealing with government agencies, but not to the private sector.

U.S. Copyright Law of 1976: This law stipulates that it is a federal offense to reproduce copyrighted materials, including computer software, without authorization.

Electronic Communication Privacy Act of 1986: The ECP Act updated the Federal Wiretap Act of 1968 and is sometimes referred to as the Wiretap Act. This law specifies that it is a crime to own any electronic, mechanical, or other device used primarily for the purpose of surreptitious interception of wire, oral, or electronic communication. This law does not apply to communication within an organization, such as email between employees.

Computer Security Act of 1987: This law mandated that the National Institute of Standards and Technology (NIST) and U.S. Office of Personnel Management (OPM) create guidance on computer security awareness and training based on functional organizational roles. In response, the NIST created the Computer Security Resource Center (http://csrc.nist .gov/index.html).

U.S. Copyright Law of 1995, amendment: This amendment protects the transmission of a digital performance over the Internet, making it a crime to transmit something for which you do not have proper authorization.

National Information Infrastructure Protection Act of 1996: This law established penalties for interstate theft of information.

U.S. Copyright Law of 1997 (No Electronic Theft Act): This addition to the copyright act creates criminal penalties for copyright infringement even if the offender does not benefit financially.

Digital Millennium Copyright Act of 1998: This legislation placed the United States in conformance with international treaties that prevail in other countries. It provides changes in three areas: protection of copyrighted digital works, extensions of copyright protection by 20 years, and the addition of criminal penalties and fines for attempting to circumvent copyright protections. In addition, it provides for copy protection for the creative organization and structure of a database, but not the underlying general facts in the database, requires that "Webcasters" pay licensing fees to recording companies, and limits Internet service providers' (ISPs') copyright infringement liability for simply transmitting information over the Internet.

Children's Online Protection Act of 2000: This law requires Web sites targeting children younger than age 14 to obtain parental consent before gathering information on children. Regulations related to this legislation issued by the Federal Trade Commission underwent significant revision in 2012 and are available for review at http://ftc.gov/opa/2012/12/coppa.shtm.

USA Patriot Act of 2001: This act gives federal officials greater authority to track and intercept communications for law enforcement and foreign intelligence purposes. With this act, law enforcement agencies now require fewer checks to collect electronic data.

Homeland Security Act of 2002: This act established the Department of Homeland Security as an executive department of the United States. It also expanded and centralized the data gathering allowed under the Patriot Act.

Cyber Security Enhancement Act (CSEA) of 2002: This act was passed along with the Homeland Security Act and reduced privacy by allowing an ISP to voluntarily hand over personal information from its customers to a government agency. Previously, a warrant was required to access such information (SANS Institute, 2004).

Controlling the Assault of Non-Solicited Pornography and Marketing Act of 2003 (CAN-SPAM Act): This act establishes a framework of administrative, civil, and criminal tools to help U.S. consumers, businesses, and families combat unsolicited commercial email or spam.

Computer Fraud and Abuse Act (CFAA) of 1984, amended in 2008: This law specifies that it is a crime to access a federal computer without authorization and to alter, destroy, or damage information or prevent authorized access. The 2008 amendment clarified a number of the provisions in the original section 1030 and criminalized additional computer-related acts. For example, a provision was added that penalizes the theft of property via computer that occurs as a part of a scheme to defraud. Another provision penalizes those who intentionally alter, damage, or destroy data belonging to others; this part of the act covers such activities as the distribution of malicious code and denial-of-service attacks. Finally, Congress included in the CFAA a provision criminalizing trafficking in passwords and similar items (U.S. Department of Justice, Computer Crime and Intellectual Property Section, 2010).

Identity Theft Enforcement and Restitution Act of 2008: This act lowers the bar for what is considered punishable identity theft crimes, thereby making it easier for prosecutors to bring charges against cybercriminals. It also makes it easier for identity theft victims to be compensated, even for costs that are indirectly associated with the harm incurred from the theft.

Since 2008, with the exception of the HIPAA changes in the Health Information Technology for Economic and Clinical Health (HITECH) Act, the federal government has not enacted significant legislation dealing with cybercrime. A comprehensive bill that failed to obtain a super-majority in the U.S. Senate focused on cybersecurity for the nation's infrastructure (U.S. Senate Committee on Homeland Security & Governmental Affairs, 2012). Since that event, additional bills have been introduced. H.R. 624: Cyber Intelligence Sharing and Protection Act passed the House of Representatives in April 2013 and was sent forward to the Senate. This bill provides for the sharing of certain cyberthreat intelligence and information between the intelligence community and cybersecurity entities (Govtrack.us, 2013). As of June 2013, this bill has not passed the Senate. The House version of the Bill and current status can be seen at http://www.govtrack.us/congress/bills/113/hr624/text#. Current federal legislation does not provide for a comprehensive approach to cybersecurity, however, this is a hot issue and future bills can be anticipated.

Protection of Computer Data and Systems

Healthcare agency procedures can help to protect the privacy and confidentiality of data as well as the safety and security of the entire system. In addition, steps that individual healthcare providers take are also important in maintaining data security. Agency responsibilities include protecting data from unauthorized use, destruction, or disclosure, and controlling data input and output. Individuals are also responsible for protecting the privacy, confidentiality, and integrity of data.

To protect data from unauthorized use, destruction, or disclosure, agencies should take the following steps:

1. Develop and maintain an ongoing risk assessment process for the institution and the specific units within the institution.
2. Develop ongoing educational programs to ensure that users understand their responsibilities.
3. Restrict access to data on a need-to-know basis by requiring passwords, personal identification numbers, and/or callback procedures.
4. Develop and enforce encoding and encrypting procedures for sensitive data.
5. Audit access (viewing) and transactions (modifying) activities. Routinely review these records and follow up on any questionable activity.
6. Develop biometric methods such as electronic signatures, fingerprints, iris scans, or retina prints to identify users.
7. Protect systems from natural disasters by locating them in areas safe from water and other potential physical damage.
8. Develop backup procedures and redundant systems so that data are not lost accidentally. In many cases when a hospital backs up the network file servers or other hospital servers it does not back up an individual local hard drive; instead, the individual is responsible for developing a system to back up these data.
9. Develop and enforce policies for both preventing and dealing with risky behavior and breaches of security.
10. Store only needed data.
11. Dispose of unneeded printouts by shredding.
12. Develop alerts that identify potentially inaccurate data such as a weight of 1200 lbs. or a blood pressure of 80/130 mm Hg.

To manage data responsibly, you should:

1. Avoid distractions and other factors that may result in data entry errors.
2. Develop a consistent process to ensure that you are on the right screen and recording the correct data. For example, always look at the patient's name before entering data on a new screen.

3. Refuse to share a password or sign in with another person's password.
4. Attend implementation/orientation classes and clearly understand institutional policies and procedures.
5. Keep the monitor screen and data out of view of other people.
6. Develop passwords that include numbers and letters that are not easy to identify.
7. Keep your own password and means of access to data secure.
8. Do not use one password or version of a password for several different systems.
9. Report unusual computer activity and potential breaches of security.
10. Encourage patients to understand their rights to privacy and confidentiality.
11. Keep harmful materials such as food, drink, and smoke away from computers.

Tools for Protecting Your PC/Mobile Device

Most healthcare agencies store information on mainframes or servers and have policies for protecting these data. However, portable or mobile devices, such as smartphones and tablets, and smaller computers such as PCs and laptops, in place throughout the institution and are much more difficult to monitor. With the increased connectivity that prevails today, many of these devices are connected to a local area network (LAN), thereby creating an intranet. In addition, many of these institutional devices have access to the Internet.

Personal mobile devices such as smartphones and tablets are rarely produced with the hardware and software security applications necessary to safely receive or transmit patient data. Therefore, it is imperative that healthcare institutions assume responsibility for ensuring that patient data are stored only on secure devices. Institutions do this by providing secure devices in the clinical settings and developing policies and procedures related to the use of personal devices.

In today's connected world there is some inevitable overlap in personal and professional communication. For example, an email requesting a volunteer to work an extra shift may be sent to a personal email account. Many healthcare providers check their work email from home. The following sections focus on ways to protect your personal computer and other devices. Protecting these devices now is not only advantageous to you, but also decreases the risk to healthcare institutions and other healthcare providers.

Antivirus Software

Computer viruses are malicious software programs that replicate themselves as they spread from one computer to another. They carry a code that can destroy files, damage hardware, and/or launch an attack on other computers. Often the user is not aware of the virus and its infection of the computer until the damage is done. Antivirus software scans the computer, email, and downloaded files to identify and disable viruses. Several companies produce and sell this type of software. Students should check whether free versions are available from their university, ISP, or a software company before purchasing any of these programs.

The majority of new computers come with antivirus software. There is wide variation as to when this software expires and will no longer receive automatic updates. Sometimes the coverage is a trial version that remains valid for only a few weeks or months. New viruses, however, are being developed and spread every day. Therefore, when installing new antivirus software, make sure that you configure this software to obtain regular updates and perform scheduled scans of your computer. Updates require that your computer be able to access the Internet and download new files from the vendor for your antivirus software. Most antivirus software programs will alert you when your subscription for updating is running out and new software must be obtained. An increasing number of antivirus software vendors are bundling anti-spyware software with the antivirus software.

Even with regular software updates a new virus can infect a computer. Always watch for alerts from your Internet service provider, employer, university, and/or software vendor concerning virus issues. Also watch for symptoms of an infected computer. **Box** 1 lists common symptoms that can indicate that a virus has infected your computer.

Box   1 Selected Symptoms of a Virus and/or Spyware

- Anti-spyware or virus software is turned off.
- Computer performance slows or freezes.
- Files or folders disappear.
- Frequent firewall alerts about an unknown program or process trying to access the Internet.
- Hard drive quickly becomes filled.
- New or different browser icons appear.
- Programs launch on their own.
- Recurring pop-up ads.
- Emails that were never sent bounce back or other email-related problems.
- The hard drive light is constantly lit.
- The Windows Control Panel Add or Remove Program includes new program(s).
- Inability to access the Web site of antivirus software companies.
- The computer makes unusual sounds, especially at random.
- The Internet home page changes even when reset.

Anti-Spyware Software

By definition, a spyware program is a type of computer software designed to install itself on your computer and then send personal data back to a central service without your permission or knowledge. Spyware secretly obtains the information by logging keystrokes, recording Web browsing history, and scanning documents on the computer's hard drive.

Adware is a specific type of spyware designed to collect data for targeted advertisements directed to your computer. As this type of software is becoming more powerful, there is increasing concern about the amount and type of personal data collected by many well-known companies without the knowledge of Internet users. Given the large number of people who search the Internet for health information, collecting these kinds of data raises important issues.

Cookies are small pieces of data that a Web site puts on your computer. They usually consist of a string of characters that identifies you to the site—something like an account number. Cookies can be useful and make the Internet more efficient by storing your preferences. In most cases, first-party cookies do not send personal information back to a central server, but third-party cookies can track Web sites that you visit and report those visits to other third-party Web sites. Of increasing concern is a specific type of cookie call a Flash cookie. This uses Adobe's Flash player technology to store information about your online browsing activities. When you delete or clear cookies from your browser Flash cookies are not deleted. As a result they are often referred to a "super cookies." Anti-spyware software identifies and deletes spyware but is often not able to delete super cookies.

Firewall

A firewall is a piece of hardware or a software program that secures the interactions between an organization's inside network of computers and the external computer environment. It achieves this goal by blocking access to the internal computer network from those outside the network and by blocking internal computers from accessing the Internet or select aspects of the Internet. By blocking external access to internal computers, a firewall can prevent a hacker or malicious software from gaining access to an internal computer. It can also prevent these types of problems from persisting on an internal computer and spreading to others.

If you are accessing a home network, such as a wireless network in your home, be sure that the firewall also protects the home network. To access the firewall in Windows, go to **Start**, **Control Panel**, and **Security**. The Windows operating system will also let you select specific programs that can access your computer or access the Internet from your computer. For example, automatic updates that are part of your antivirus and anti-spyware software, as well as Windows updates, require free passage through the firewall.

Web Browser Security Settings

Because your browser is often your interface to the Internet, it is important that you configure it to ensure your computer's protection as well as your own privacy. For example, you may want to protect your computer from a site downloading malware on your computer by blocking cookies from being stored on the computer and by protecting your credit card information while shopping online.

The first step in keeping your browser secure is keeping it current. If possible, set your browser to check for updates on a regular basis. This includes checking for updates for any add-ons or apps installed with your browser. It is helpful if your selected browser provides a Web page for checking to confirm that your browser is current and that installed add-ons are also up-to-date.

Protecting your computer and your privacy can include a phishing filter, a pop-up blocker, notification that a Web site is trying to download files onto your computer, and/or notification if a program's digital signature is current and correct when you are trying to download a program or files. Your browser can also provide you with a 128-bit secure encrypted connection for activities such as interaction with online financial or medical sites. With this protection, when you visit a Web site whose URL starts with "https," a small padlock symbol appears in the browser window. This symbol indicates that the Web site is a secure site and uses a digital certificate to notify you of that fact. A few trusted Certification Authorities (CAs) issue those certificates.

Because each browser has its own procedure for configuration, you must search to find the appropriate settings; use the browser's help section to ensure that you have provided your computer with the highest level of protection possible. Key settings include:

- Pop-up blocker
- Do Not Track
- Third-party cookies
- Saving history and cookies
- Overall level of security

As you select each of these settings there are three points that you should carefully evaluate:

1. What are you opening or blocking? For example, if you select **InPrivate Browsing,** your browser won't retain cookies, your browsing history, search records, or the files you downloaded after you log off; however, when you are connecting to the Internet you are connecting to other computers that can record that information. Your ISP, your employer (if using a work computer), and the sites you have visited can track your Internet activities.

The InPrivate Browsing function can be a useful function for an abused client searching for support services on a home computer and trying to keep that search history from the abuser. It would not protect an employee whose employer is tracking their Internet use.

2. How effective is the setting? For example, if you select **Do Not Track** you are instructing the Web site that you visit to not track your activities. There is no way to ensure that the site will honor your request.

3. How will this setting affect your computer use and functionality? For example, you may decide to block third-party cookies. Remember, the difference between a first-party cookie and a third-party cookie is not in the coding of the cookies, but rather is determined by the context of a particular visit. If a cookie is associated with the page you are viewing, it's a first-party cookie. For example, if you visit CNN.com and the cookie is from CNN it is a first-party cookie. A cookie from a different domain is a third-party cookie. As described above, companies often use third-party cookies to track your activity across sites and then use this information to support targeted advertising. However, you can use these same cookies to support more effective Internet searching. You, the user, must evaluate the advantages and disadvantages of third-party cookies.

NOTE: Some sites that you might access, such as your school's email or course management software for online courses, may require that you turn on certain settings. For example, Blackboard—a type of course management software for delivering online and Web-enhanced courses—requires that cookies and JavaScripts be enabled for that Web site. This means you need to turn that feature on for only that Web site.

Password Protection

You can control who has access to the files on your computer by password-protecting the computer itself. In addition, individual files can be password-protected. However, be sure to use good password design to ensure that others cannot easily decipher it and make sure that you can remember it. Password-protected files are lost if you can't remember the password. They *cannot* be reset by IT like your network password nor can Microsoft reset Office program passwords. **Box   2** provides guidelines on creating strong passwords.

If you are using a home wireless network like those that many broadband services provide, make sure the network is password-protected. If it is not, anyone with a wireless card can access the connection when they are in range.

Box   2 Do's and Don'ts for Creating Strong Passwords

- Use at least eight characters (more is better).
- Combine letters and symbols.
- Use both lower and uppercase letters.
- Select characters from the whole keyboard.
- Use a different password for each application.
- If you write the passwords down, store them in a safe place, not on your computer or device.
- Change passwords regularly.
- Do not use your password on public computers.
- Do not use your name, Social Security number, birth date, or other data that can be associated with you. This includes names spelled backward.
- Avoid dictionary words or common communication abbreviations such as lol or icu.
- Avoid sequences such as qwer or 8765.
- Do not repeat characters.
- Create a complete sentence and use the first letter from each word with numbers in the middle.

User Guidelines for Protecting Your PC

While some of the same guidelines related to safety and security of mainframes and servers are important for the PC, additional guidelines apply when you want to protect the PC system and its data. Often individuals are concerned about the privacy of information on their computers and about the information that others may access on their PCs when they use the Internet. The following is a summary of action steps to protect the data on your PC.

Protecting Your Email

- Install a virus checker to routinely scan your computer's hard drive(s).
- Configure your virus checker to scan email and downloaded files as they come in.
- Scan email attachments before opening them. Do *not* set your mail to automatically open attachments.
- Do not open email or attachments if you do not know the sender.

- If you use a filter to screen your mail, remember to empty the mailbox where the junk mail goes.
- Use whatever methods your email system provides to protect your mail from snooping, tampering, and forgery.
- Report spam or suspicious email to your ISP.

Downloading Files

- Download data only from reputable systems; those systems regularly check their files for viruses.
- Configure your virus software to scan files before downloading them.
- Scan data storage devices that others have given to you before opening the files.

Using the Internet

- Install and routinely update your firewall.
- Do not stay connected to the Internet for long periods when you are not using it.
- If others have access to your computer, install a password so that they can't sign on to the Internet without your permission.
- Do not tape passwords on the wall or hide them under your keyboard.
- Use only reputable cloud and online backup services.

Protecting Your Computer

- Use an approved surge protector to protect the PC. Remember: A power strip may not provide surge protection.
- Load only sealed software from a reputable vendor.

Protecting Your Data

- Regularly perform system backups and rotate the storage media that you use for the backup procedure.
- If data are lost due to a virus, scan the backups before installing them to ensure you are not reinstalling the virus.
- Do not store backups in the same area as the computer; store them offsite or use a fireproof safe.
- Store sensitive data on a secure external hard drive and store the hard drive in a locked area.
- Connect the secure external hard drive to the computer only as needed. Remember to disconnect the external hard drive when you are finished using it.

- Name sensitive files cryptically.
- Hide important files by using utilities and avoid using the computer hard drive by storing sensitive data on other devices such as external hard drives, memory sticks, and so forth.
- Use a cross cut paper shredder when disposing of paper documentation.
- Label storage media such as CDs and DVDs so that you can easily determine the contents of a disc.
- Eliminate old or unnecessary backup files.
- Remove sensitive data before taking a computer in for repair or, better yet, don't store sensitive data on the hard drive (C).

Protecting Your Personal Identity

- Examine the implications of your email address listings and the use of other information that you provide to your online service provider and other Internet resources.
- Never give out personal information on a chat room or online discussion group and never "click here" to provide personal information to an email saying there is an issue with your account.
- Many online companies ask permission to use your email address to send future information. Check No if you do not want that service and want to request that they do not pass your email address on to others.
- Use the secure server when you are given that option. A secure server provides additional protection when you are sending private information such as a credit card number via the Internet.
- Keep one credit card for Internet use only. Some credit card companies will issue a second card with a different number for just this purpose.
- Look for the padlock icon. When you are sending data to a private Internet site, such as your bank, look for the padlock icon on the screen. This icon signifies that your data are encrypted and you are on a secure site. Alternatively, look for the http to be https, which means you are accessing a secure server.
- Know the policies related to using email. If you transfer messages from your ISP to your own computer, you may have more privacy protection than if you leave those messages on the provider's server.

These guidelines provide a foundation for securing your computer and your privacy. However, Internet-related applications used on a computer change rapidly as the use of the Internet continues to expand. **Table** 5 provides additional resources for protecting your computer. **Table** 6 provides resources for protecting children on the Internet. **Box** 3 provides general guidelines for protecting mobile devices, such as smartphones and tablets. Always remember that there is no such thing as total privacy or security when using the Internet.

TABLE 5 RESOURCES FOR PROTECTING YOUR COMPUTER AND YOURSELF ONLINE	
Resource	URL
U.S. Department of Homeland Security: United States Computer Emergency Readiness Team	http://www.us-cert.gov/cas/tips/
Federal Trade Commission: OnGuard Online	http://www.onguardonline.gov/ Can be viewed in both English and Spanish.
Microsoft Safety & Security Center	http://www.microsoft.com/security/default.aspx
Stanford School of Medicine Information Security Services*	http://med.stanford.edu/irt/security/

* Many schools in the health professions have Web sites similar to this one. You might want to check with your school to see if they have information posted that deals with this topic.

TABLE 6 RESOURCES FOR PROTECTING CHILDREN ONLINE	
Resource	URL
Center for Schools and Communities: Protecting Children Online	www.center-school.org/pko/resources.php
Federal Bureau of Investigation	www.fbi.gov/stats-services/publications /parent-guide
Federal Trade Commission	www.onguardonline.gov/topics/protect-kids-online
Goodwill Community Foundation, Inc.	www.gcflearnfree.org/internetsafetyforkids
National Cyber Security Alliance	www.staysafeonline.org/teach-online-safety/
South Carolina Information Sharing & Analysis Center	https://sc-isac.sc.gov/content/protecting-children-online

Box   3 Protecting Your Mobil Device and Your Privacy

1. Review the product manual, the manufacturer's Web site, and the Internet service provider's (ISP's) Web site for specific directions and advice related to privacy and security settings.

2. Check for updates on a daily basis and install patches to the operating system when they are available.

3. Install security software that includes antivirus, firewall, and spam blocker functionality.

4. Use your device's auto-lock feature and functionality. For example, set the auto-lock to take effect within minutes of your last activity.

5. Create a strong password and/or pin. Do not use your birthdate, house number, last four digits of your Social Security number, or numbers in sequence such as 1234 or 2468 as a pin number.

6. Use unique passwords for applications with sensitive data.

7. Avoid using sensitive apps on open or public networks.

8. Do not share your device with others, especially if you cannot use separate passwords.

9. Turn off your Wi-Fi and Bluetooth when they are not needed. Do not set Wi-Fi to connect automatically.

10. Do not include sensitive personal information such as your driver's license number, Social Security number, password, or account numbers in text messages.

11. Only download mobile applications from authorized application stores like the Apple App Store or Google Play, formerly known as the Android Market.

12. Notify your ISP immediately if your mobile device is missing.

13. Install software or an app that can wipe out information remotely.

14. Keep your mobile device backed up so you do not hesitate to wipe out information if you cannot locate your mobile device.

15. Install a tracking application to locate your device if it is missing or stolen.

Providing Patient Care via a Computer

While most healthcare providers are well aware of the computer as a tool for documenting care and managing the healthcare record, that application is only part of how providers use computers to deliver care and communicate with patients, clients, and consumers. Three key areas of health care now dealing with major security issues in electronic communication include: (1) the electronic transmission of **personal health information (PHI)**, (2) the use of the Web as a health information and emotional support resource, and (3) the use of email between healthcare providers and clients.

Federal Regulations and Guidelines for the Exchange of Personal Health Information

In their early days, healthcare information systems consisted of individual computer systems designed for specific functions. Over time, however, healthcare providers began networking these islands of information. The early networks were simple. For example, one of the early interfaces involved connecting the lab to the clinical units so that the lab could quickly transmit lab results back to the clinical unit.

Today, a group of federal agencies and private organizations are building a Nationwide Health Information Network (NwHIN) to securely exchange electronic health information on a national level. These organizations are developing and implementing the work standards, services, and policies necessary to establish a comprehensive network of interoperable network systems. The NwHIN is transmitting clinical, public health, and personal health information, with the goal of improving decision making by ensuring that health information is available when and where it is needed (U.S. Department of Health and Human Services, Office of the National Coordinator for Health Information Technology, n.d.).

With the increasing use of technology and interconnectivity, local institutions and others serving a number of healthcare institutions store medical information in a variety of computer databases. Needless to say, the security of personal health data within an electronic health system is a growing concern. The Health Insurance Portability and Accountability Act of 1996, which has as its goal the simplification of the administrative processes used to transmit electronic health information, represented a major step forward in building the needed security standards, policies, and procedures. In passing HIPAA, Congress required the U.S. Department of Health and Human Services to adopt national standards for electronic healthcare transactions, code sets, unique health identifiers, and security. This law established standards for transmitting health data, including standards for transmitting PHI. These standards were the first federal regulations to address privacy and security of PHI. In December 2008, the U.S. Department of Health and Human Services' Office of the National Coordinator for Health Information Technology released *The Nationwide Privacy and Security Framework for Electronic Exchange of Individually Identifiable Health Information*, which reads in part:

The principles below establish a single, consistent approach to address the privacy and security challenges related to electronic health information exchange through a network for all persons, regardless of the legal framework that may apply to a particular organization. The goal of this effort is to establish a policy framework for electronic health information exchange that can help guide the Nation's adoption of health information technologies and help improve the availability of health information and health care quality. The principles have been designed to establish the roles of individuals and the responsibilities of those who hold and exchange electronic individually identifiable health information through a network (p. 1).

The principles underlying this document are summarized in **Table** 7.

The Health Information Technology for Economic and Clinical Health (HITECH) Act was enacted as part of the American Recovery and Reinvestment Act of 2009 and it modified HIPAA through several provisions that strengthened the civil and criminal enforcement of the HIPAA rules. The complete suite of HIPAA Regulations includes:

- Transactions and Code Set Standards
- Identifier Standards
- Privacy Rule
- Security Rule
- Enforcement Rule

Additional details about these standards and rules are located at http://www .hhs.gov/ocr/privacy/hipaa/administrative/combined/index.html.

The Web as a Health Information and Emotional Support Resource

Web sites are fast becoming a major—if not *the* major—source of health information for the general public. Discussion boards and social media sites on the Internet are also emerging as a major source of emotional support for those facing difficult health issues.

Patient Portals and Electronic Communication with Patients

While many healthcare providers have been hesitant to use electronic communication with patients, increasing numbers of patients are demanding this form of communication. Patients are especially interested in scheduling appointments, renewing prescriptions, obtaining test results, and getting the answers to health questions. Healthcare providers are often reluctant to engage in such

Principle	Definition
TABLE 7 PRINCIPLES OF THE NATIONWIDE PRIVACY AND SECURITY FRAMEWORK FOR ELECTRONIC EXCHANGE OF INDIVIDUALLY IDENTIFIABLE HEALTH INFORMATION	
Individual Access Principle	Individuals should be provided with a simple and timely means to access and obtain their individually identifiable health information in a readable form and format.
Correction Principle	Individuals should be provided with a timely means to dispute the accuracy or integrity of their individually identifiable health information and to have erroneous information corrected or to have a dispute documented if their requests are denied.
Openness and Transparency Principle	There should be openness and transparency about policies, procedures, and technologies that directly affect individuals and/or their individually identifiable health information.
Individual Choice Principle	Individuals should be provided a reasonable opportunity and capability to make informed decisions about the collection, use, and disclosure of their individually identifiable health information.
Collection, Use, and Disclosure Limitation Principle	Individually identifiable health information should be collected, used, and/or disclosed only to the extent necessary to accomplish a specified purpose(s) and never to discriminate inappropriately.
Data Quality and Integrity Principle	Individuals and entities should take reasonable steps to ensure that individually identifiable health information is complete, accurate, and up-to-date to the extent necessary for the person's or entity's intended purposes and has not been altered or destroyed in an unauthorized manner.
Safeguards Principle	Individually identifiable health information should be protected with reasonable administrative, technical, and physical safeguards to ensure its confidentiality, integrity, and availability and to prevent unauthorized or inappropriate access, use, or disclosure.
Accountability Principle	These principles should be implemented, and adherence assured, through appropriate monitoring, and other means and methods should be in place to report and mitigate nonadherence and breaches.

NOTE: The information in this table was developed for U.S. Department of Health and Human Services, Office of the National Coordinator for Health Information Technology (2008). Nationwide privacy and security framework for electronic exchange of individually identifiable health information. Retrieved from http://www.healthit.gov/sites/default/files/nationwide-ps-framework-5.pdf

communication because of concerns related to security issues, malpractice, and the possibility they will not be able to manage the increased workload.

However, financial incentives within HITECH strongly support electronic communication with patients. As a result, increasing numbers of healthcare providers are now beginning to use electronic communication with patients as part of their electronic health record applications. Safe use of electronic communication, however, requires educating both the healthcare provider and the healthcare recipient.

Summary

Storing data and exchanging these data via the computer system raise several privacy, security, and confidentiality concerns. This chapter focused on issues related to confidentiality and privacy of data, as well as methods to ensure the integrity of data, software, and hardware. Securing computers and the data they store pose a challenge both for large healthcare information systems and for individuals using PCs. The development of the Internet has created a whole new level of opportunity—and a source of concern. Protecting the privacy of patients and the integrity of their health-related data depend on carefully crafted laws and on educating both the provider and the consumer of health care. Fundamental to that security is understanding the applications and activities necessary to secure your personal computer, related devices, and data.

References

American Health Information Management Association (AHIMA) e-HIM Workgroup on Assessing and Improving Healthcare Data Quality in the HER (2007). Assessing and improving EHR data quality. *Journal of AHIMA, 78*(3), 69–72.

American Medical Association (AMA) (2007). *The Patriot Act: Implications for physicians.* Retrieved from http://www.ama-assn.org/ama/pub/physician-resources/legal-topics /patient-physician-relationship-topics/patriot-act.page

Burke, L. & Weill, B. (2005). *Information technology for the health professions.* Upper Saddle River, NJ: Prentice Hall.

Computer Crime and Intellectual Property Section (CCIPS), U. S. Department of Justice (2010). *Prosecuting computer crimes.* Retrieved from http://www.justice.gov/criminal /cybercrime/docs/ccmanual.pdf

Daniel, M. (2012, January 8). Collaborative and Cross-Cutting Approaches to Cybersecurity. [The White House Blog]. Retrieved from http://www.whitehouse.gov/blog/2012/08/01 /collaborative-and-cross-cutting-approaches-cybersecurity

Federal Trade Commission (2012a). *Medical identity theft.* Retrieved from http://www .consumer.ftc.gov/articles/0171-medical-identity-theft

Federal Trade Commission (2012b). *Child identity theft.* Retrieved from http://www .consumer.ftc.gov/articles/0040-child-identity-theft

Federal Trade Commission (2012c). *Tax-related identity theft.* Retrieved from http://www .consumer.ftc.gov/articles/0008-tax-related-identity-theft

Govtrack.us (2013) H.R. 624: Cyber Intelligence Sharing and Protection Act. Retrieved from http://www.govtrack.us/congress/bills/113/hr624#

Jenkins, M. K. (2011). Medical records of the rich and famous—A huge risk. [Web log]. Retrieved from http://www.physicianspractice.com/blog/medical-records-rich-and-famous-%E2%80%94-huge-risk

Johnson, M. E. (2009). *Data hemorrhages in the healthcare sector.* Retrieved from http:// fc09.ifca.ai/papers/54_Data_Hemorrhages.pdf

Medical Information Board (MIB) (n.d.). *The facts about MIB.* Retrieved from http://www .mib.com/facts_about_mib.html

National Academy of Sciences, Computer Science and Telecommunications Board (1997). Privacy and security concerns regarding electronic health information. In *For the record: Protecting electronic health information* (chapter 3). Retrieved from http://www .nap.edu/openbook/0309056977/html/54.html

Ornstein, C. (2009, May 11). Farrah Fawcett 'under a microscope' and holding onto hope. *Los Angeles Times.* Retrieved from http://www.latimes.com/entertainment/news/la-et-fawcett-interview11-2009may11,0,5790379.story?page=1

Privacy Rights Clearinghouse (2012a). *Privacy Rights Clearinghouse fact sheets.* Retrieved from https://www.privacyrights.org/privacy-rights-fact-sheets

Privacy Rights Clearinghouse (2012b). *Fact sheet 8: Medical records privacy.* Retrieved from http://www.privacyrights.org/fs/fs8-med.htm

Privacy Rights Clearinghouse (2012c). *Children's online privacy: A resource guide for parents.* Retrieved from http://www.privacyrights.org/fs/fs21-children.htm

SANS Institute (2004). *Federal computer crime laws.* Retrieved from http://www.sans.org /reading_room/whitepapers/legal/federal-computer-crime-laws_1446

U.S. Department of Health and Human Services (HHS) (2011, July 7) University of California settles HIPAA privacy and security case involving UCLA Health System facilities. *Press release.* Retrieved from http://www.hhs.gov/news/press/2011pres/07 /20110707a.html

U.S. Department of Health and Human Services (HHS), Office of the National Coordinator for Health Information Technology (2008). *Nationwide privacy and security framework for electronic exchange of individually identifiable health information.* Retrieved from http://www.healthit.gov/sites/default/files/nationwide-ps-framework-5.pdf

U.S. Department of Health and Human Services (HHS), Office of the National Coordinator for Health Information Technology (n.d.). The Nationwide Health Information Network, Direct Project, and CONNECT Software. [Software] Available from http:// www.healthit.gov/policy-researchers-implementers/nationwide-health-information -network-nwhin40

U.S. Department of Health and Human Services, Office of Civil Rights (2008). *The HIPAA privacy rule's right of access and health information technology* (HIT). Retrieved from http://www.hhs.gov/ocr/privacy/hipaa/understanding/special/healthit/index.html

U.S. Senate Committee on Homeland Security & Governmental Affairs (2012). *Senate rejects second chance to safeguard most critical cyber networks*. Retrieved from http://www .hsgac.senate.gov/media/majority-media/senate-rejects-second-chance-to-safeguard -most-critical-cyber-networks-

Exercises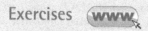

■ **Objectives**

1. Apply ethical concepts in making decisions about the use of computers in commonly encountered situations.
2. Clarify your personal attitude about the ethical use of computer hardware and software.
3. Recognize computer-related criminal behavior.

■ **Activity**

Your personal ethics are your foundational principles for making decisions about how you will and will not conduct yourself. Health professionals are guided by the ethical code of their specific discipline. In the table below you will see several examples of these codes. As a professional in health care, you will be expected to make ethical decisions about the appropriate use of computers.

1. Start this exercise by first reviewing the codes of ethics posted on the following sites. As you review these documents, pay special attention to the sections on privacy and confidentiality.

Professional Association	URL for the Code of Ethics
American Medical Association (AMA)	http://www.ama-assn.org/ama/pub/physician-resources/medical-ethics/code-medical-ethics.page?
American Nurses Association (ANA)	http://nursingworld.org/MainMenuCategories/EthicsStandards/CodeofEthicsforNurses
Association for Computing Machinery (ACM)	http://www.acm.org/about/code-of-ethics
American Medical Informatics Association (AMIA)	http://www.amia.org/about-amia/ethics/code-ethics
National Association of Social Workers (NASW)	http://www.socialworkers.org/pubs/code/code.asp
International Medical Informatics Association (IMIA)	http://www.imia-medinfo.org/new2/node/39
American Occupational Therapy Association (AOTA)	http://www.aota.org/Practitioners/Ethics/Docs.aspx
American Health Information Management Association (AHIMA)	http://www.ahima.org/about/ethicscode.aspx

In addition to these sites be sure to explore both the Dashboard and Professional Categories located at http://ethics.iit.edu/ecodes/.

2. Beside each situation below, place a check by the term(s) that best reflects your opinion of the behavior of the individual. Provide your reasoning for each of your answers using both the ethical codes of conduct and the information on computer crimes presented in this chapter.

   a. John and Beth are both enrolled in the same section of a computer class. The textbook is expensive so they decide to split the cost and share the required textbook. The book includes access to a Web site; however, it is designed so only one account can be established. They elect to establish one account in Beth's name and share the password.

   John: Ethical___ Unethical___ Computer crime___
   Beth: Ethical___ Unethical___ Computer crime___

   b. At the end of the term John and Beth decide to sell the textbook and the Web access to a student, Robert, who will be taking the course next term. While the password for the Web site can be changed the user name cannot be changed.

   John: Ethical___ Unethical___ Computer crime___
   Beth: Ethical___ Unethical___ Computer crime___
   Robert: Ethical___ Unethical___ Computer crime___

   c. Susan is a senior nursing student recovering from a respiratory infection that required treatment with antibiotics. She was glad to be told by her doctor that by Wednesday she will no longer be contagious. This term Susan is taking Nurs 401. In this course the students are expected to obtain their clinical assignment on Tuesday and prepare for a 6-hour clinical on Wednesday. Susan asks a classmate, Betty, who is assigned to the same clinical unit to check her assignment and to make notes of the information she will need to research, such as the patients diagnosis, significant diagnostic tests, medications, and treatment. The classmate is glad to be of help because they often work together in preparing for clinical and helping each other on the clinical unit.

   Susan: Ethical___ Unethical___ Computer crime___
   Betty: Ethical___ Unethical___ Computer crime___

   d. Betty was surprised to discover that she was not able to help Susan. On Tuesdays nursing students are only able to access the patient(s) on the hospital computer system that are included in their assignments. Betty notifies Susan, who then calls her clinical instructor, Dr. H. Ple to explain her dilemma. Dr. H. Ple comes to the clinical unit and prints off the information. She blacks out the patient's name and gives the printout to Betty who takes it back to Susan.

Susan: Ethical___ Unethical___ Computer crime___
Betty: Ethical___ Unethical___ Computer crime___
Dr. H. Ple: Ethical___ Unethical___ Computer crime___

e. James is assigned to an observational learning experience in a busy emergency department. Five patients from a multiple-car accident have just been admitted and more are expected. James is observing Dr. Smith who is gloved and intubating one of the patients. All of the staff are currently busy caring for the other patients. Dr. Smith's beeper emits a series of beeps. Dr. Smith explains to James that the beeper is hospital issued and requires a password. She tells James that the series of beeps indicates an emergency and she asks James to use her password to sign on and read the text message aloud. James signs in with Dr. Smith's password and reads the message, which includes a patient's name, a brief description of the problem, and requests for a return call STAT.

James: Ethical___ Unethical___ Computer crime___
Dr. Smith: Ethical___ Unethical___ Computer crime___

f. Brian is creating a Web page and finds a terrific background graphic on another page. He copies the background to use on his page. He also includes at the bottom of the page in small print a link acknowledging the source of the background.

Brian: Ethical___ Unethical___ Computer crime___

g. Several healthcare providers are collaborating on an important research study that includes a review of the patient's history, a guided interview, and a computed tomography scan (CT) for each patient participating in the study. The hospital Institutional Board of Review (IRB) has given permission for data collection of the patients' health history via computerized patient records for patients who have signed the informed consent forms. In the past, once the IRB approval was obtained, the principal investigator (PI) sent a list of names of the co-investigators to the IT department to establish their research-related computer accounts. The co-investigators would then review the patient's records and set up the data collection format for each patient. Late Friday afternoon the PI receives a memo explaining that the IT procedures have been changed and the accounts will not be established until the co-investigators have signed the appropriate forms and received training that includes the policies and procedures for using the computerized patient records. Several patients have already been scheduled for interviews and CTs on

Saturday. All of the co-investigators currently have access to the computerized record for these patents via their hospital responsibilities. The PI and co-investigators decide to use their hospital access and deal with the change in procedures on Monday.

> PI: Ethical___ Unethical___ Computer crime___
> Co-investigators: Ethical___ Unethical___ Computer crime___
> IT Department: Ethical___ Unethical___ Computer crime___

h. Terri has taken 21 credits this term and has had a very difficult time keeping up. In 48 hours she must turn in a term paper on the use of computers in health care. She discovers an online term paper titled *The Use of Computers in Rural Hospitals*. The outline is perfect so she uses the paper as a "jumping off point," making significant revisions to the paper. Since she does not cite a specific section of the paper she does not include the paper in her references.

> Terry: Ethical___ Unethical___ Computer crime___

i. Dr. Bob is teaching a computer course. The university purchased a site license for 25 copies of the software he is distributing to students. However, 25 students are registered for the course. Dr. Bob gives each of the students an account and sends in a purchase request for additional copies so he will also have access. A week later he receives a call from the purchasing department informing him that the site licenses are only sold in bundles of 25 and cost $500. Dr. Bob decides to wait a week to determine if any students drop the course. If a student does drop the course Dr. Bob plans to use the student's account for his own access.

> Dr. Bob: Ethical___ Unethical___ Computer crime___

j. James is completing his senior year as a nursing student in a BSN program. A patient he cared for a few weeks ago obtained his email address from the online university directory and sent him an email. In the email the patient discussed new and potentially serious symptoms and asks that James keep his concerns confidential. James believes the symptoms may indicate a life-threatening situation. He forwards the email to the charge nurse on the unit where the patient was treated and to the senior resident involved in the patient's care.

> James: Ethical___ Unethical___ Computer crime___

3. Based on what you've learned during this exercise, create a personal code of ethics to guide your activities in the classroom and the clinical environment. Save the file as **Chap13-Exercise1-LastName** and submit it to your instructor as directed.

EXERCISE 2 Discovering Personal Information on the Internet

■ **Objectives**

1. Gain an appreciation of how much personal information is available on the Web.
2. Understand the options you have and do not have to protect your private information.

■ **Activity**

1. Select three different Internet search engines. Use each of the them to search for your professor's name on the Internet. Then search for your name. Note what information you find in each case—what did you learn about your professor and yourself. Did you find information that could be misleading or that was not accurate?
2. Professor Emeritus John W. Hill, JD, PhD http://kelley.iu.edu/Accounting /faculty/page12887.cfm?ID=8277 is a recognized legal expert with a distinguished academic record. Review his bio and then use each of the three search engines to see what else you can learn about this man. Now read the post at http://urbanlegends.about.com/od/government/a/Blue-Cross-On -Medicare.htm. This is an example of how a professional's reputation and credentials can be stolen and used on the Internet.
3. Using only your name or phone number, search the Internet to determine if you can locate a street map or picture of your home and/or your parent's home. Note how long it takes you, from the time you start this search until the time you find the information.
4. Using your Word application, write a brief paper explaining what you learned from this exercise and your reaction to this information. Consider whether any of the information you found would be helpful or would hinder you if you were applying for a position in health care.
5. Save this file as **Chap13-Exercise2-LastName**. If you are using a discussion board, respond to the discussion thread on this exercise.

EXERCISE 3 Copyright and Plagiarism

■ **Objectives**

1. Describe copyright restrictions and the fair use doctrine.
2. Identify the difference between copyright violations and plagiarism.
3. Identify methods for adhering to copyright law when writing a research paper.

■ **Activity**
1. Copyright and plagiarism
   a. Access and review the following Web sites:
      ■ www.copyright.gov/ Explore the different links, then review the document located at *Copyright Basics (en Español)* and view the video located at *Taking the Mystery Out of Copyright.*
      ■ http://www.lib.utsystem.edu/copyright/. Complete the tutorial.
      ■ http://www.libraries.psu.edu/psul/lls/students/using_information.html.
   b. Evaluate the follow scenarios to determine if there is a copyright violation and/or plagiarism. If there is plagiarism or a violation, how should it be handled? Remember that while any one activity may represent both plagiarism and a copyright violation, plagiarism and copyright violation are different issues.
      1. A student is writing a term paper and asks another student to review the paper. The second student makes several revisions from correcting spelling to rewriting sentences. The second student does not add any new citations. In a couple of places she does add examples that clarify some of the concepts included in the original version of the paper. The second student is not paid for the review but does offer to review future papers for pay.
      2. Three students are reading a newly published article written by one of their previous professors. They are surprised and pleased to discover that the professor has acknowledged them at the beginning of the article. The acknowledgement simply states that their insights have been helpful in writing the article. However, in reading the article, each student has discovered a short section (two to three paragraphs) that is almost a direct quote from a term paper previously submitted to the professor.
      3. As a class assignment a student is writing a manual that includes a list of terms with definitions. The student searches the Internet for these terms and uses definitions from a combination of sites when creating each definition.
      4. A student is writing a paper on Meaningful Use and includes a table posted on a government Web site demonstrating how the Centers for Medicare & Medicaid Services are calculating financial incentives. While the Web site for the Centers for Medicare & Medicaid Services is included in the references (http://www.cms.gov/Regulations-and-Guidance/Legislation/EHRIncentivePrograms/index.html) the table does not include a citation.
2. Based on your review of the Web sites and the analysis of the scenarios, answer the following questions:
   a. What is a copyright?
   b. What is fair use?

c. What is the public domain?

d. What are the guidelines for including information in a term paper so as to be in compliance with the copyright law?

e. What is the difference between copyright violation and plagiarism?

3. Type your answers to the questions and save this file as **Chap13-Exercise3-LastName**. Submit it as directed by your professor.

EXERCISE 4 Preventing Computer Crime

■ Objectives

1. Apply information about computer crimes to prevent these crimes in commonly encountered situations.

2. Understand current laws as they apply to computer crimes.

■ Situation

During the school year you are living in a dorm with a roommate. Your roommate has an older computer that is having technical problems. There are only a few more weeks left in the term and you know your roommate does not have the money to buy a new computer. Several times he has asked to use your laptop for both school and personal use. How can you configure your computer to protect your privacy? What guidelines or rules should you require your roommate to observe when he is using your laptop?

■ Activity

1. Review the materials that are available within this chapter and the Web sites listed.

2. Search for Web sites that provide information about protecting your computer, data, and software.

3. Describe the steps you would take to configure your computer and its browser(s) to protect your privacy.

4. Write a set of rules/guidelines that can be used for the next few weeks.

5. Describe how you would ensure that your guidelines are followed.

6. Save this document as **Chap13-Exercise4-LastName**. Submit it as directed by the professor.

Assignments

ASSIGNMENT 1 Copyright—A Student Government Educational Piece

■ Situation

Several professors at your university are concerned about increasing incidences of copyright infringement. Many of the faculty believe that the ease with which students can cut and paste information from a Web site or an online document has exacerbated this problem. In response to their concerns the faculty senate asked the student government association to create a video that can be posted on YouTube dealing with the many challenges that students face while researching online databases and the Internet. You are on the student government board of directors and a part of a student group assigned the task of developing the video.

■ **Directions**

1. Use the following URLs or find other sites to help you develop your video content:

   http://www.templetons.com/brad/copymyths.htm
   http://www.bitlaw.com/copyright/fair_use.html
   http://library.stanford.edu/using/copyright-reminder/copyright-law-overview
   http://vcuhvlibrary.uhv.edu/studyguides/copyright.htm
   http://www.plagiarism.org/

2. Create a script for the video and an announcement of the video. Use an appropriate variety of fonts, bold, italics, underlining, graphics, or other formatting features so that the announcement has an eye-catching format. If directed by your professor, develop the video and upload it to YouTube.

3. Save the file as **Chap13-Assign1-LastName** and submit as directed by your professor.

ASSIGNMENT 2 Tablet Use Guidelines

■ **Situation**

The School of Health Professions Learning Lab faculty and staff received a grant to purchase tablets for student use in the clinical area. The tablets include references that can be used to research medications, diagnoses, diagnostic tests, standards of practice, and other clinical materials. These tablets can also be used to access the university network for recording notes and sending emails. Due to their cost, the tablets must be rotated among two groups of students, and therefore, must be checked out the afternoon before clinical and returned the afternoon of clinical.

As the graduate assistant working with the principal investigator (PI) for this grant your charge is twofold: (1) prepare a handout with guidelines on maintaining the safety and security of the tablets and (2) prepare a short presentation to the tablets including these guidelines. This presentation will be shown during the students' orientation.

■ **Directions**

1. Prepare a list of potential issues and the guidelines, you can give to the PI for review. Make sure to format the guidelines appropriately, including any graphics that might reinforce them.

2. Save this file as **Chap13-Assign2a-LastName**. Submit your list of safety and security issues and your guidelines to your instructor.
3. Because you know that most of the students are already oriented to PowerPoint, create a short PowerPoint presentation that can be shown during student orientation. This presentation will be loaded on the laptops to provide a quick reference. Make sure to follow the guidelines for quality presentations. Set the program to run automatically.
4. Save this presentation as **Chap13-Assign2b-LastName** and submit it to your professor.

ASSIGNMENT 3 Issue Critique

■ **Directions**
1. Select one of the following statements to critique:
   a. Information posted on a public discussion board is public domain and can be freely used in total as long as it is properly cited.
   b. The patient owns their data. Therefore, when those data are stored in an electronic health record, each patient has a legal right to know the name of each person who has accessed their record.
   c. Electronic health records are more secure than paper health records, therefore the more sensitive the data (i.e., history of drug and alcohol abuse, AIDS diagnosis, and mental health status) the more important it is that these data be stored electronically.
   d. If the policies and procedures for using the computer system in a healthcare setting create a safety risk for a patient, you should meet the patient's needs and then deal with the policy issues.
2. Write a one- to two-page paper identifying points that support or refute the statement you select. Conclude by stating your position and reasons for that position.
3. Save the file as **Chap13-Assign3-LastName** and submit it to your professor.

NOTE: If this course has an online component, this assignment can be part of a discussion forum requirement, where you will support or refute the statement selected and respond to classmates' posts.

ASSIGNMENT 4 Guidelines for Electronic Communication

■ **Situation**
You are the school nurse in a local public school with 428 students in grades K to 6. Today the principal asked to meet with you. At that meeting the principal stated

that she is concerned about both the tone and content of electronic communication between:

   a. Teachers
   b. Teachers and Parents
   c. Students and Teachers
   d. Students

In her judgment some of the emails are aggressive in tone (maybe even bullying) and some seem to divulge confidential information concerning students' health and learning problems. She has asked that you research this problem and provide a set of recommendations to address it.

■ Directions

1. Develop a list of references and resources you will use in developing the recommendations.
2. Create an outline of the key topics you would address within the recommendations.
3. Using the information you have found create a flyer with a set of guidelines for the children in grades 4 to 6.
4. Run a readability index on the document to be sure that the reading level is appropriate for the students.
5. Save the file as **Chap13-Assign4-LastName**. Submit the references, resources, outline, and the guidelines to your professor.

The Electronic Medical Record: Efficient Medical Care or Disaster in the Making?

Dale Buchbinder

You are the Chief Information Officer (CIO) of a large health care system. Medicare has mandated that all medical practices seeking Medicare compensation must begin using electronic medical records (EMR). Medicare has incentivized medical practices to place electronic medical records in their offices by giving financial bonuses to medical practices that achieve certain goals. These EMR systems are supposed to allow communication between practitioners and hospitals, so medical information can be rapidly transferred to provide more efficient medical care. The EMR will enable physicians to allow access to the records of their patients by other providers. Eventually these records are supposed to be easily accessed so any physician or hospital will have complete medical information on a patient.

The physician practices in your health care system have been mandated to use the Unified Medical Record System (UMRS). The UMRS was designed by a central committee; all hospital-owned physician practices have been mandated to use the system. As part of the incentives, Medicare will add dollars back to each practice when they meet goals for reaching meaningful use (MU). MU has been defined by the U.S. Department of Health and Human Services (n.d.) as "using certified electronic health record (EHR) technology to:

- Improve quality, safety, efficiency, and reduce health disparities
- Engage patients and family
- Improve care coordination, and population and public health
- Maintain privacy and security of patient health information."

It is a step-by-step system requiring "electronic functions to support the care of a certain percentage of patients" (Jha, Burke, DesRoches, Joshi, Kralovec, Campbell, & Buntin, 2011, p. SP118).

One of the hospitals in your system has many primary care and specialty practices; however, the UMRS system was designed primarily for the primary care practices. The committee that developed UMRS did not take into account the needs of the specialty practices, which are significantly different from the primary care practices. This issue has been brought to the forefront by several medical specialists who have stated UMRS is not only cumbersome, but also extremely difficult to use. UMRS also does not give the specialist the information he needs. Specialists noted that after UMRS was implemented, it took them approximately 10 to 15 minutes longer to see each patient. Since an average day for a specialist consists of seeing between 20 and 25 patients, adding 10 to 15 minutes per patient adds 200 to 250 additional minutes, or 3 to 4 hours more each day. And, the physician cannot see the same number of patients each day. In reality, this represents a 30% decrease in productivity because of the amount of time it takes to use UMRS. Now the specialist office schedules constantly run significantly later than they should, and patients become unhappy and impatient. Several of the specialists reported that a number of patients have gotten up and left without being seen. In short, the mandate to use UMRS has impacted the efficiency and productivity of the subspecialists and specialists, further decreasing revenues for the system.

In addition, all of the physicians have complained the UMRS does not communicate well with other electronic medical record systems, or even the hospital's own patient information systems. There is no real integration of the medical databases as intended, levels of meaningful use are unclear, and in some areas, difficult to achieve, again because the UMRS was tailored to primary care practices' prescribing patterns. Specialists, particularly surgeons, do not write a large number of prescriptions. Surgeons have been mandated to write electronic prescriptions to reach meaningful use; however, in many cases this is not appropriate for surgical patients.

All of these issues and concerns were reported to the central committee that created UMRS in response to federal mandates and financial incentives. The committee responded it cannot modify the system to make it more friendly to specialists and subspecialists, despite the fact that procedures performed by the subspecialists account for substantial revenues. Revenues are down and the morale of the specialists and subspecialists has plummeted to the point that many are talking about taking early retirement or leaving the system. Still, the committee refuses to fix the problems. Since you are the CIO of the entire health care system, the situation is now in your hands. What will you do?

Discussion Questions

1. What are the facts in this situation?
2. What are three organizational issues this case illustrates?
3. What are the advantages and pitfalls to EMR? Should all types of practices be required to use the same system? What role should physicians play in selecting and developing an EMR system to fit their individual practices? Provide a rationale for your responses.
4. Is there a way to bring consensus and standardize the EMR systems without alienating productive physicians who bring large revenues to the hospital? How can the dilemma of inefficiency and patient dissatisfaction be prevented? Create and present a plan for how EMR could be implemented in a system with multiple types of practices. Be sure to address the issues of physician specialty, productivity, and satisfaction, as well as patient satisfaction.
5. What steps should the CIO take in the future to prevent these types of issues from occurring again? Provide your reflections and personal opinions as well as your recommendations and rationale for your responses.

ADDITIONAL RESOURCES

Borkowski, N. (2011). *Organizational behavior in health care* (2nd ed.). Sudbury, MA: Jones and Bartlett.

Buchbinder, S. B., & Buchbinder, D. (2012). Managing healthcare professionals. In S. B. Buchbinder & N. H. Shanks (Eds.), *Introduction to health care management* (2nd ed., pp. 211–247). Burlington, MA: Jones & Bartlett.

Cresswell, K., Worth, A., & Sheikh, A. (2012). Integration of a nationally procured electronic health record system into user work practices. *BMC Medical Informatics and Decision Making, 12,* 15.

Fallon, L. F., & McConnell, C. R. (2007). *Human resource management in healthcare: Principles and practices.* Sudbury, MA: Jones and Bartlett.

Hudson, J. S., Neff, J. A., Padilla, M. A., Zhang, Q., & Mercer, L. T. (2012). Predictors of physician use of inpatient electronic health records. *American Journal of Managed Care, 18*(4), 201–206.

Jha, A., Burke, M., DesRoches, C., Joshi, M., Kralovec, P., Campbell, E., & Buntin, M. (2011). Progress toward meaningful use: Hospitals' adoption of electronic health records. *The American Journal of Managed Care, 17*(12 Spec No.), SP117–SP124.

Mandl, K., & Kohane, I. (2012). Escaping the EHR trap—The future of health IT. *The New England Journal of Medicine, 366*(24), 2240–2242.

Morrison, E. E. (2011). *Ethics in health administration: A practical approach for decision makers* (2nd ed.). Sudbury, MA: Jones and Bartlett.

Shen, J. J., & Ginn, G. O. (2012). Financial position and adoption of electronic health records: A retrospective longitudinal study. *Journal of Health Care Finance, 38*(3), 61–77.

Tiankai, W., & Biedermann, S. (2012). Adoption and utilization of electronic health record systems by long-term care facilities in Texas. *Perspectives in Health Information Management,* 1–14.

U.S. Department of Health and Human Services. (n.d.). *EHR incentives & certification: Meaningful use definition & objectives.* Retrieved from http://www.healthit.gov /providers-professionals/meaningful-use-definition-objectives

Yan, H., Gardner, R., & Baier, R. (2012). Beyond the focus group: Understanding physicians' barriers to electronic medical records. *Joint Commission Journal on Quality & Patient Safety, 38*(4), 184–191.

The Case of the Snoopy PA

Dale Buchbinder

You are the Chairperson of Surgery and manager in charge of a group of physician assistants and nurse practitioners who are responsible for the care of patients on a busy surgical service at Downtown General Hospital (DGH). Barbara Newman, a surgical physician assistant (PA), comes to your office and states that Bill Smith, another surgical PA, had called her over to his computer. On the screen were the test results of a coworker, the unit secretary on the main surgical floor. She had been admitted to the ER, and her lab results were positive for illicit substances.

Barbara was distressed at this situation. She knew the unit secretary's personal medical history had been violated. Not only was this unethical because Bill was not involved in her care, but also he had shared this information with several coworkers, a major HIPAA* violation. The hospital compliance officer has confirmed the computer login trail is clear. Bill was, indeed, viewing records he had no clinical need to be viewing. Your next action is to confront Bill with this situation and see what his response will be.

---

* "The Health Insurance Portability and Accountability Act (HIPAA) of 1996 is one effort to protect patient information in the modern hospital. According to the Office of Civil Rights (2012), a portion of HIPAA was designed to protect patient privacy and confidentiality in secure environments, particularly through electronic transactions. The regulations protect medical records and other individually identifiable health information, whether on paper or in electronic or oral communications. Key provisions of these new standards include rules and regulations regarding: access to medical records; notice of privacy practices; limits on the use of personal and medical information; prohibitions on marketing; stronger state laws; confidential communications; and provisions for patient complaints in case they feel their rights have been violated" (Zeiler, 2012, p. 345).

Discussion Questions

1. What are the facts of this case?
2. What is the nature of the organizational behavior problem?
3. Which theory or theories do you believe best explain the behavior of the PA's coworker?
4. Is this a case of a violation of patient privacy and a HIPAA* (See definition above.) violation? What additional data, if any, would the Chairperson need to collect to document this violation?
5. Should the PA be verbally warned, suspended from work for a period of time, or terminated? Provide a rationale for your responses.
6. What types of legal and ethical issues are identified in this case study?
7. What kind of clinical and financial impacts do you think the PA's behavior could have on the hospital if it went unchecked?
8. Do you think this problem was addressed appropriately? Provide your reflections and personal opinions as well as your recommendations and rationale for addressing this problem.

Role Play

The Chairperson: One student is the Chairperson of the department. It is that student's job to confront the PA and see what his response is. Keeping in mind the Discussion Questions and Additional Resources for this case, how can the Chairperson ensure safe, effective patient care and maintain patient privacy?

Bill, the Surgical PA: One student is the snoopy PA. It is that student's job to convince his boss and Chairperson that he didn't do it, that he logged into the computer and someone else used it. Keeping in mind the Discussion Questions and Additional Resources for this case, how can he defend his behaviors?

ADDITIONAL RESOURCES

Borkowski, N. (2011). *Organizational behavior in health care* (2nd ed.). Sudbury, MA: Jones and Bartlett.

Buchbinder, S. B., & Shanks, N. H. (Eds.). (2012). *Introduction to health care management* (2nd ed.). Burlington, MA: Jones & Bartlett.

Centers for Medicare and Medicaid Services (CMS). (2012). *Medical privacy of protected health information: Information for Medicare fee-for-service health care professionals.*

Retrieved from http://www.cms.gov/Outreach-and-Education/Medicare-Learning
-Network-MLN/MLNProducts/downloads/SE0726FactSheet.pdf

Fallon, L. F., & McConnell, C. R. (2007). *Human resource management in healthcare: Principles and practices.* Sudbury, MA: Jones and Bartlett.

Morrison, E. E. (2011). *Ethics in health administration: A practical approach for decision makers* (2nd ed.). Sudbury, MA: Jones and Bartlett.

Office of Civil Rights (OCR). (2003). *Summary of the HIPAA privacy rule.* Retrieved from http://www.cms.gov/Regulations-and-Guidance/HIPAA-Administrative
-Simplification/HIPAAGenInfo/Downloads/HIPAALaw.pdf

Office of Civil Rights (OCR). (n.d.). *Health information privacy.* Retrieved from http://www.hhs.gov/ocr/privacy/

Patterson, K., Grenny, J., McMillan, R., & Switzler, A. (2004). *Crucial confrontations.* New York, NY: McGraw-Hill.

Patterson, K., Grenny, J., McMillan, R., & Switzler, A. (2011). *Crucial conversations: Tools for talking when stakes are high* (2nd ed.). New York, NY: McGraw-Hill.

Zeiler, K. (2012). Ethics and law. In S. B. Buchbinder & N. H. Shanks (Eds.), *Introduction to health care management* (2nd ed., pp. 333–350). Burlington, MA: Jones & Bartlett.

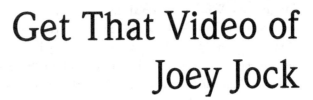

Get That Video of Joey Jock

Nancy H. Shanks

The Phixemup Clinic and Rehabilitation Facility was a world-renown orthopedic practice. With more than 25 years of treating professional football, basketball, and baseball players, as well as world-class golfers, it had built a reputation for being "the place" for treatment of all types of athletic injuries. Many "weekend warriors" and budding amateur athletes utilized the Clinic for their treatment and rehab.

The Phixemup physicians were extremely well regarded as providing cutting-edge treatment and getting people back to their sports quickly. The founding physician, Dr. Phixemup, had led the practice, making it able to attract the best and the brightest young physicians, many of whom trained as his fellows. Several had recently been hired to meet the increasing demands of this busy practice.

Many of the Phixemup staff, including the practice manager, had worked there since the Clinic first opened, but several had recently retired. This placed significant pressure on HR to fill these positions, to bring on additional support staff for the new physicians, and to staff for the increasing demand that would result. The HR Department was trained to expedite the hiring and training process, but got behind in the training of new hires.

Joey Jock, the handsome, heartthrob star quarterback of the NFL Pittsfield Pistols injured his anterior cruciate ligament (ACL) in spring training. He was immediately scheduled for assessment with Dr. Phixemup, who quickly scheduled surgery in an effort to address the problem and get him into rehab and back on the field as soon as possible.

Word of Joey's visit, surgery, and rehab spread like wildfire through the staff. Susiecue was one of the new hires in the IT Department. She was a computer whiz, but had no health care background. She was enamored with Joey and just couldn't resist taking a peek at his medical record and gleaning some personal information. When she learned that he had a follow-up appointment the next day, she thought it would be fun to have her camera phone ready. Without getting permission, she took a short video of Joey hobbling through the office on his crutches. Susiecue was really pleased with the footage and decided to post it online. It immediately went viral!!! Later that night, Susiecue got a call at home from the new practice manager telling her to be in at 8:00 am sharp the next morning to meet with her and the HR Director.

Discussion Questions

1. What are the privacy issues associated with medical records? Who should have access to them? What should be the rationale for such access?
2. What responsibility does the practice have for ensuring that the staff has been trained about confidentiality, privacy, and HIPAA issues?
3. Given the practice's clientele, should extra precautions be taken to shield and protect the privacy of celebrities being treated at Phixemup?
4. What are the legal and ethical issues associated with Susiecue's actions?
5. What penalties may the practice face for HIPAA violations?
6. What other liabilities may result from the case?
7. What is likely to have happened to Susiecue at the morning meeting?
8. What should management do to prevent these types of breaches from happening again? Should they give certain patient records "VIP" status or should all records be handled the same way? Should access to medical records be monitored?

ADDITIONAL RESOURCES

Buchbinder, S. B., & Shanks, N. H. (Eds.). (2012). *Introduction to health care management* (2nd ed.). Burlington, MA: Jones & Bartlett.

Conn, J. (2010). Holes in the fence? In an era of expanding electronic interchange, privacy protections are being put to the test. *Modern Healthcare, 40*(47), 26–28.

Conn, J. (2011). The burden of privacy? Demands placed by proposed privacy rule could outweigh patient benefits. *Modern Healthcare, 41*(24), 30–32.

Frauenheim, E. (2008). Snooping into health records often unnoticed. *Workforce Management, 87*(9), 6.

Halamka, J. D. (2009). Your medical information in the digital age. *Harvard Business Review, 87*(7/8), 22–24.

McWay, D. C. (2010). *Legal and ethical aspects of health information management* (3rd ed.). Clifton Park, NY: Cengage.

Mir, S. S. (2011a). HIPAA privacy rule: Maintaining the confidentiality of medical records, part 1. *Journal of Health Care Compliance, 13*(2), 5–14.

Mir, S. S. (2011b). HIPAA privacy rule: Maintaining the confidentiality of medical records, part 2. *Journal of Health Care Compliance, 13*(3), 35–44 +.

Vogt, N. (2004). Privacy compliance: Are we sending mixed messages? *Journal of Health Care Compliance, 6*(6), 34–35.

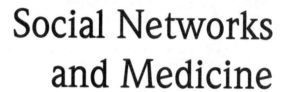

Social Networks and Medicine

Kevin D. Zeiler

The Riverbend Hospital, a hospital located in a rural area of the state, recently purchased laptops for all employees of the hospital system, as well as emergency responders. The goal of the purchase was to streamline medical treatment and information in real time so that patients could receive more timely care. The program has been in place for just over three months with most of the employees feeling that the new system has been a real time-saver. However, a recent leak of patient information has put the program in jeopardy.

Because the laptops are provided with Internet access, many of the hospital's employees have been using them for personal web browsing, social network updating, etc. Ambulance crews have been uploading photos from crash sites, shootings, etc., so that physicians and nurses can be made aware of the mechanism of injury and such. However, an employee in the system recently posted some of those photos to a social network site that many members of the local community share, and it has brought to light an abusive relationship that is taking place in the small community. The photos clearly show the patient and most, if not all, citizens in the small community know her. Furthermore, other providers have started to post comments about her treatment, follow-up care, and other medical conditions. The female patient is currently seeking legal advice and the future of the hospital's new computer system has been compromised.

Discussion Questions

1. You are the director of the electronic record delivery program at Riverbend and want to see the program continue. However, given the above circumstance, what Act must you rely on to guide you in this process? What does this Act say about the use of electronic medical information?
2. What legal options does the patient have as it pertains to this case?
3. If the program does survive, what can you do as the director to ensure that something like this does not happen again?

ADDITIONAL RESOURCES

Buchbinder, S. B., & Shanks, N. H. (Eds.). (2012). *Introduction to health care management* (2nd ed.). Burlington, MA: Jones & Bartlett.

Furrow, B. R., Greaney, T. L., Johnson, S. H., Jost, T. S., & Schwartz, R. L. (2008). *Health law: Cases, material and problems* (6th ed.). St. Paul, MN: Thomson-West.

Pozgar, George. (2012). *Legal aspects of health care administration* (11th ed.). Sudbury, MA: Jones & Bartlett.

White, A. (2010). *Hospitals and providers: Five guidelines for HIPAA compliance in social media.* Retrieved from http://lovell.com/healthcare/hospitals-and-providers-five-guidelines-for-hipaa-compliance-in-social-media/

Index